Making Healing Remedies with Honey and Propolis

Carolyn K Gibson

ISBN-10: 1979926883
ISBN-13: 978-1979926881

DEDICATION

We thank God the Father for the bees and all the wonders of nature. We worship God the Father but not his creations.

CONTENTS

DISCLAIMER

This book is for information only. It is not to be taken as medical advice.
It is not meant to be a substitute for consulting with your healthcare
provider.
Caution: If you are allergic to bees you could be allergic to honey or
propolis. You could have an allergy to any of the herbs listed.

To err is human. Every attempt has been made to make sure all
information is accurate. The author and publisher are not responsible for
errors.

1 Introduction

The Lord has provided many natural remedies for us, herbs, honey and propolis.

As with all natural remedies they are difficult to verify in the test tube. Natural remedies are subject to the weather, where the plant was grown, or in the case of honey and propolis where the bees harvested these products, which particular property the bees were gathering for the benefit of the hive and what time of the year.

Longtime bee keepers here in the United States are just now discovering the healing properties of honey and propolis.

Europe and Asia have been using these bee products for centuries.

This book is not meant to provide all possible remedies or bore you with all possible research data.

This is meant to get you started and you should continue your own research. Nothing works like trial and error.

I have been making herbal remedies since the '70s and just started using honey and bee propolis in recent years.

My main research for honey and propolis include:
www.greenmedinfo.com

National Institute of Health
A part of the U.S. Department of Health and Human Services, NIH is the largest biomedical research agency in the world.
www.nih.gov

Propolis Power Plus by Carson Wade with Joan A. Friedrich, PH.D
User's Guide to Propolis, Royal Jelly, Honey, and Bee Pollen by C. Leigh Broadhurst, Ph.D.
The New Honey Revolution by Ron Fessenden, MD, MPH
The Honey Prescription by Nathaniel Altman: Medical Writer and Researcher
Two Million Blossoms by Kirsten S. Traynor, M.S.
Many herb books and classes
My personal experience

The NIH website has many recipes for making honey and propolis remedies. Some of their recipes contain ingredients you may not recognize and question if they are natural, petroleum jelly being the main one.
Other ingredients you may not recognize are:
Propylene Glycol: a natural gas
Sorbitol: from corn
Sodium Sterate: from coconut oil
Sodium Laureth Sulfate: from coconut oil

Making Healing Remedies with Honey and Propolis

Glycerin: can be plant based or petroleum based**, research your source**
Titanium Dioxide: from ilmenite ore

All remedies do not work for all people. There are some remedies with propolis and some with honey or herbs. Which works for you may is a matter of personal experience and which that you have on hand. It is not like the Lord gave us only one remedy and if it is not available, tough luck. He put many different healing remedies all over the world. As you experiment, seeing is believing.

Natural remedies are not miracle cures that you can use one time and expect miraculous results. Just like the drug store medicines they need to be applied or taken several times a day.

Sometimes your immune system has been so compromised you will need to see a doctor and get a prescription.

Sometimes, nothing works.

Maybe you have been under a lot of stress, overworked or over obligated.
Your body will demand rest. If you getting sick are the only way to get rest, so be it.

Nutrition, exercise, cleanliness, rest and recreation may be the answer to the problem, and no amount of natural healing is going to take the place of these.

More research is showing our immune system begins in the gut. You may need to start taking probiotic.

This is not a religion. Natural remedies are a first step in healing; if it is not working see your medical professional.

2 Healing with Honey

The Lord made the bees and the flowers, and the bee makes the honey. The bees gather nectar from the flowers; they bring it up back up from their stomachs, combine it with their spit to change the nectar into honey.

All honey is not equal in medical benefits. Lighter colored honey will generally taste better but does not offer the best medical benefits. The honey foraged from wildflowers would be more effective than a one crop honey. Honey foraged from conifer trees would be even more effective. The more variety of flowers the bee forages from the better the medical and nutritious benefits. The exception would be the Manuka honey and Revamil which has the most medical benefits.

Ancient cultures used honey therapeutically and many ancient texts prescribe honey for sores, wounds and sore eyes. It is valued all over the world as medicine except the United States. For some reason the United States does not value the research of other nations.

In the 1930's honey was scientifically proven to be an effective antimicrobial. In 1989 and 1992 there were many other studies providing proof of Honey's medical value.

Honey is so effective for skin wounds, that in the UK they have a medically approved honey that is used in the hospitals called Medihoney (which is the Manuka honey) and in the Netherlands they have one called Revamil (which the bees are raised in a closed greenhouse to guarantee their source of nectar). Of course these honeys are very expensive. They are the only ones allowed in the hospitals. These honeys have been Gamma irradiation to kill all microbes and spores. The antibacterial potency of these honeys has been verified.

Manuka honey is rated by its' antibacterial potency. UMF (Unique Manuka Factor). Medical professionals in New Zealand use Manuka honey for its' medical benefits with a rating of at least 10 UMF. If you are paying the big bucks for Manuka honey check its' UMF rating.
Go to the web site below for further information.
http://www.honey.bio.waikato.ac.nz

 Regular raw, wildflower honey will work in most cases even though their antibacterial potency has not been verified. For serious infections you would definitely use the Manuka honey. Very serious infections will require the specially developed Manuka honey products such as gels and impregnated bandages.
Go to http://www.dermasciences.com for complete descriptions of these products. Order these products on Amazon.

Pathogens Treated with Honey: from 1992 Peter Molan's review "The antibacterial activity of honey"

Bacillus anthracis:
Anthrax
Corynebacterium diphtheria:
Diphtheria
Escherichia coli:
Diarrhea, septicemia, urinary tract infections, wound infections
Haemophilus influenzae   :
Ear infections, meningitis, respiratory infections, sinusitis
Listeria monocytogenes   :
Meningitis
Mycobacterium tuberculosis:
Tuberculosis
Pasteurella multocida:
Infected animal bites
Proteus species :
Septicemia, urinary tract infections, wound infections
Pseudomonas aeruginosa:
Urinary tract infections, wound infections
Salmonella species:
Diarrhea
Salmonella cholerae-suis:
Septicemia
Salmonella typhi:
Typhoid
Salmonella typhimurium:
Wound infections
Serratia marcescens:

Septicemia, wound infections
Shigella species:
Dysentery
Staphylococcus aureus:
Abscesses, boils, carbuncles, impetigo, wound infections
Streptococcus faecalis:
Urinary tract infections
Streptococcus mutans:
Tooth decay
Streptococcus pneumonia:
Ear infections, meningitis, pneumonia, sinusitis
Streptococcus pyodenes:
Ear infections, impetigo, puerperal fever, rheumatic fever, scarlet fever,
sore throat, wound infections
Vibrio cholera:
Cholera

More research has shown raw honey to be effective against
Helicobacter pylori and the super bug MRSA.
Keep in mind that many of these treatments require Manuka with
special honey products such as gels, impregnated dressings and honey
leather. Many of the tests were done with honey that has a UMF rating
of 15 or better. Healing was not overnight. Many weeks of treatment
are required for some ailments.

When buying honey for its medical benefits you will want raw,
unprocessed or minimal processed honey. Many bee keepers will strain
their honey to remove bee parts and other debris. Straining is different
than filtering. Filtering would also remove the pollen, which you want
to keep. However you do not want it strained to the point the pollen

has been removed. The bee keeper can control this with the size of strainer that he uses. Royal jelly added to the honey would make it even more powerful.

Honey is the second most lied about product in the US. Americans only produce 1/3 of the honey sold in America. Misleading labeling allows much honey to be sold as local or raw, or even 100% honey.

Buy raw, unprocessed honey from health food stores, farmers markets, road side stands. Check Bee Keepers websites in your area to find bee keepers in your area. Many honeys that are in the grocery stores and big box stores have been processed, have removed the pollen and some may have added corn syrup.

Honey is an effective treatment to prevent and treat all kinds of infected wounds and burns and out performs chemical based medicines. Wounds heal faster with less scarring. Ancient use of honey is now becoming proven in research to work against drug resistant bacteria and fungus. The University of Waikato Honey Research Unit adds the additional benefits of using honey for wounds is reduced inflammation, reduction in pain, and naturally sloughs off dead tissue.

Wounds that can be treated with Manuka Honey:
Serious infections may require the Medihoney products such as gels and impregnated bandages and require a qualified medical professional.
Source: Dr. Molan, director of the Honey Research Unit:
Abrasions
Amputations
Abscesses

Bed sores
Burst abdominal wounds following caesarian delivery
Cancrum oris (gangrenous ulcers of the mouth)
Cervical ulcers
Chilblains (inflamed swelling or sores caused by exposure to cold)
Cracked nipples
Cuts
Diabetic foot ulcers and other diabetic ulcers
Fistula
Foot ulcers in lepers
Infected wounds arising from trauma
Large septic wounds
Leg ulcers
Malignant ulcers
Sickle-cell related ulcers
Skin ulcers
Surgical wounds
Tropical ulcers
Varicose ulcers
Wounds to the abdominal wall and perineum

Most wounds heal best in a moist environment. A moist environment supports bacteria growth. Honey solves this problem because of its antibacterial properties.

Honey can be applied directly to infected wounds, ulceration and bedsores and burns, first, second or third degree, and then covered with a sterile cloth. It can be applied directly to abscess and will pull out the infection, leaving a hole. Continue to use the honey to heal the hole.

Using honey to heal wounds does have its problems.
It is sticky.
Depending on the temperature, the honey may become too liquefied causing it to ooze out making it difficult to keep on the wound. In this case it would be easier to use the special prepared honey dressing available with Manuka honey.
A small percentage of people may feel a temporary stinging sensation when the honey is applied to the wound.
Ground up bee pollen can be mixed in with the honey to make it thicker and stay on the wound better.

Main Antibacterial Properties of Honey
Osmosis: Cells require equilibrium. When they are put into sugar saturation, such as honey, the water in the bacteria or fungi cells seek equilibrium and basically die of dehydration. Burns and wounds could be treated with sugar solutions but these sugar solutions lack the other antibacterial properties of honey.

Acidity: Honey has a ph of 4, which is acidic. Acidity inhibits the growth of bacteria.

Hydrogen peroxide production: Honey does not contain hydrogen peroxide, but produces it when it comes in contact with body fluids around a wound in a minuscule amounts, in a continuous, slow release fashion, effective against bacteria but not harmful to the body.
We all remember hydrogen peroxide from our childhood. It was fascinating watching it foam and bubble up around our sores. For the most part it did not sting. Hydrogen peroxide does destroy bacteria on contact but will also damage skin tissue. Doctors may use it diluted on

patients or full strength to clean instruments. I use hydrogen peroxide to disinfect my kitchen counters instead of bleach.

Floral nectar: Depending on which flowers the bees have harvested there are unknown components that have antibacterial properties. Flavonoids and antioxidants are also present in different amounts depending on the flowers harvested.

Other Health Benefits
Enhances the immune system, reduces inflammation and stimulates cell growing.

Honey is both a probiotic and a prebiotic. Its antioxidant properties will vary according to the flowers it forages and the different locations it forages from.   You would need to eat 4-10 tablespoons a day to raise the antioxidant's levels in your blood. Generally speaking, darker honey has more antioxidants and a stronger flavor.

Studies have found honey to be effective against respiratory infections and more effective than dextromethorphan and diphenhydramine in relieving night time coughs.
Honey is even more effective when combined with herbs into an herb infused honey, or into herbal honey syrup, or an oxymel.

Herbal honey is not the same as a variety of honey. A variety of honey is when the bees forages one variety of plants such as almond trees, clover, orange blossoms etc. An herbal honey has herbs infused into it.

A simple herbal honey syrup is made by combining equal parts of herbal honey, herbal tincture, and a concentrated herbal tea.

Honey and Diabetics

1 tablespoon of honey has nearly the same carbohydrate (glucose-fructose) content as a medium apple.

Children and Honey

Yes, botulism spores have been found in honey. The difference is that the spores cannot grow in honey. Our immune system can deal with these microbes but an infant under 1 year may not. Botulism can cross the brain blood barrier (which can lead to meningitis) until the baby is 18 -24 months old.

Cooking and Sweetening with honey.

Honey is sweeter than sugar and less honey can be used in many recipes. However sugar has its own taste that gives the recipes a certain taste. Even though it will sweeten the recipe it will not taste the same.

 Honey taste great in herbal teas but does not do as well in coffee. Coffee is bitter and honey does not seem to offset the bitterness for me. We drink Starbucks dark roasted coffee and we drink it strong. For my taste I use 1 teaspoon of raw sugar with 1 teaspoon of honey in my coffee, or I use as much as a tablespoon of honey.
You can replace up to half the sugar with equal amounts of honey in your recipes.
When baking with honey reduce the liquids by ¼ cup for each cup of honey you are using, add ½ teaspoon of baking soda and reduce the over temperature by 25∘f.

Even though many books suggest that you may lose weight because honey is sweeter and you use less does not work for me. However, I do not crave sweets as I once did. Sugar creates a desire for more and more sugar, honey does not. The honey I am using throughout the day seems to reduce my desire for something sweet.

Honey will not ferment in the stomach as sugar does causing gas and bloating.

For honey recipes and suggestions go to:
http://www.honey.com

3 Honey Recipes

Herb Infused Honey

Ground or minced dried herbs
Equal amount of honey

Stir together and heat for 6-8 hours, keeping the temperature under 110°f -115°f.

Strain,
Bottle,
Label with the ingredients and the date.

Herb Infused Honey

Honey infused with dried herbs has a very long shelf life. Using fresh herbs will dilute the honey and will require refrigeration.

1. Mix grounded or chopped herbs with an equal amount of honey by volume (wildflower honey preferred) if using powdered herbs reduce the herbs by 1/2 as much honey.

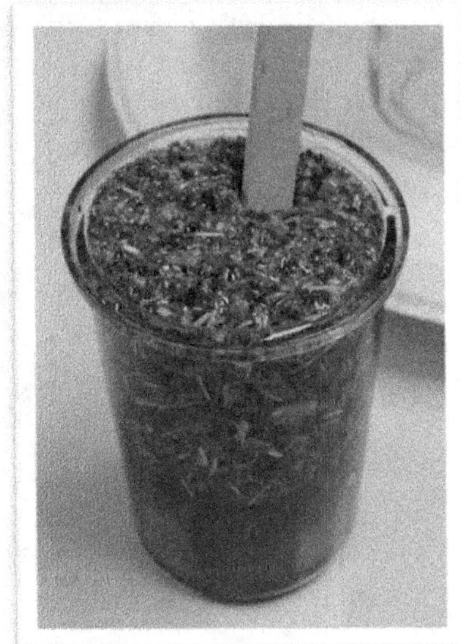

2. Place the honey and herb mixture in the top of a double boiler, or

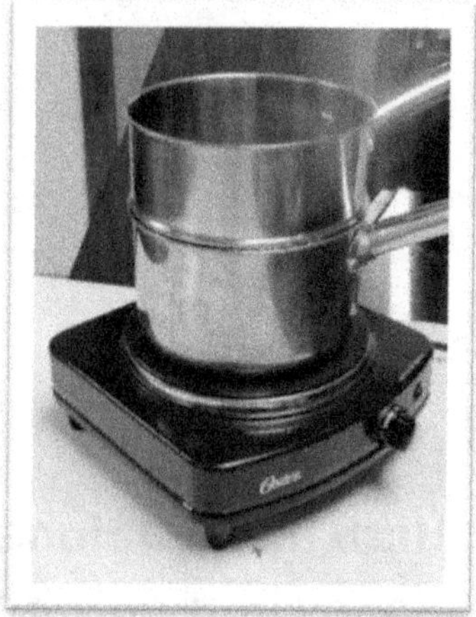

A crock pot or,

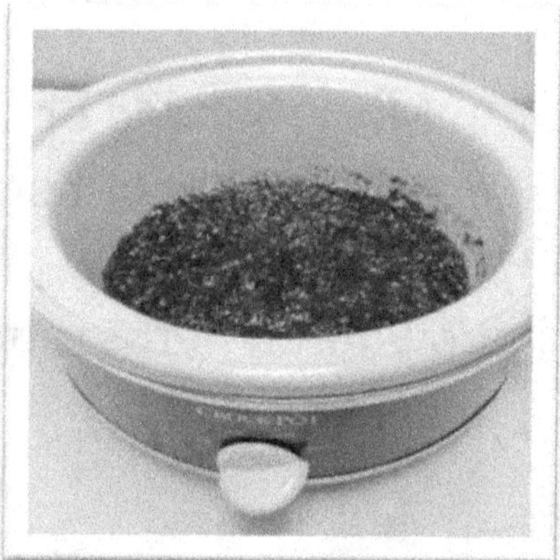

A yogurt maker will allow you to make several varieties at one time.

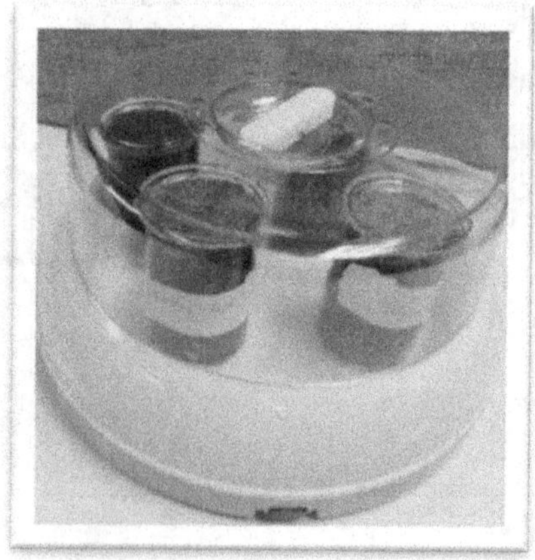

 If the honey is heated in a double boiler be sure and check the water and check the honey herb mixture to make sure the herbs are completely covered, adding more honey if necessary.

3. Strain the herbal honey while still warm with cheesecloth, muslin bag, reusable coffee filters or any other strainer.

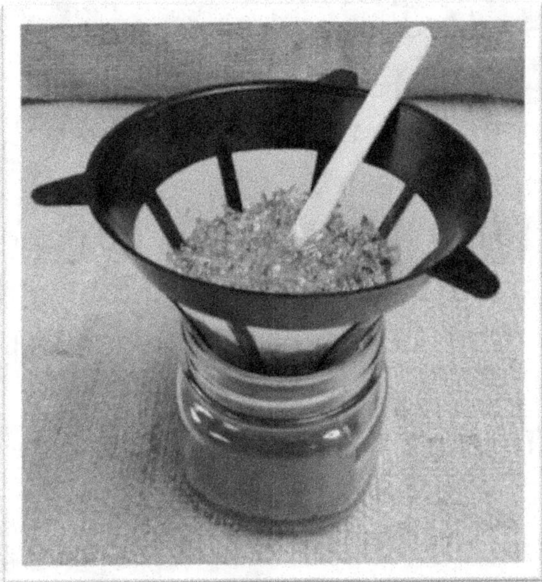

4. Pour into a glass container and cap. Label with the name of the herb, honey and the date. You can take this straight, add to hot water or herbal tea or use to make herbal syrup.

How to Make Honey Herb Syrup

2 oz. of dried herb
1 quart of water, distilled preferred
1 -2 cups of honey

1. Mix the dried herb with the water.
2. Simmer the liquid and reduce to 1 pint.
3. Strain
4. Pour the concentrated herb tea back into the pot.
5. Add 1-2 cups of honey to taste.
6. Heat only enough to mix the 2 together. Do not destroy the important properties of the honey from too much heat.
Optional: Add a few drops of essential oils such as peppermint or spearmint.
Add a little Propolis Tincture, Vodka or Brandy to help preserve your syrup.
Remove from heat, bottle and label with the name of the ingredients and the date.
Refrigerate. This should keep for several months.

Note on using herbs:
Seeds, barks and roots can normally be boiled without losing their healing benefits. Leaves and flowers are normally steeped to preserve their healing properties.
 If the herbs you are using are the leaves and flowers making an infused honey would be better. If using the seeds, bark or roots then the honey syrup would be better.

Herbal teas available in the grocery store are normally a good quality of herb. When needing a small amounts of herbs these can be used. Simply remove from the tea bag.
If you have a favorite herb tea blend, try making an Herb Infused Honey or Herbal Honey Syrup with the tea blend.

Herbs such as ginger, anise seed, thyme, oregano can easily be found in your grocery store. For long time storage, store your herbs in the refrigerator.

Elderberry Syrup

Elderberry Syrup

½ cup dried elderberries, or 1 cup of fresh
2 cinnamon sticks
5 cloves
2 cups of water, distilled preferred
1 cup of water if using fresh berries
1-2 cups of honey
1 tablespoon of lemon juice
Optional: 12 Star Anise or 1 teaspoon of Anise Seed
1 teaspoon of dried ginger or 1 tablespoon of fresh grated ginger

Anise Seed will act as both an expectorant (thins the mucus) and will help suppress the cough.

Take 1 tablespoon every hour or at least several times a day at the first sign of cold or flu, continue throughout the illness.
Use for coughs as both a cough suppressant and expectorant.
Take for coughs that produce a lot of mucus.

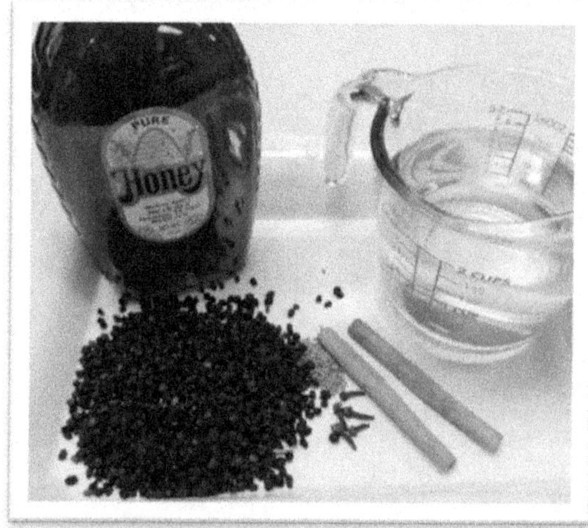

½ cup of dried elderberries
Or 1 cup if using fresh or frozen elderberries
5 cloves
2 cinnamon sticks
2 cups of water (distilled preferred) 1 cup of water if using fresh elderberries
1-2 cups of Honey
Optional: 12 Star Anise or 1 teaspoon of Anise Seed.
Star Anise and Anise Seed are different herbs.

1 tablespoon of grated fresh ginger or 1 teaspoon of the dried ginger powder
1 tablespoon of lemon juice
Small saucepan with lid, muslin cloth or other strainer

Combine the dried elderberries and other herbs with 2 cups of water, 1 cup of water if using fresh or frozen elderberries.
Cover the pan and bring to a boil and then simmer for about 20-30 minutes or until the liquid is reduced by half.

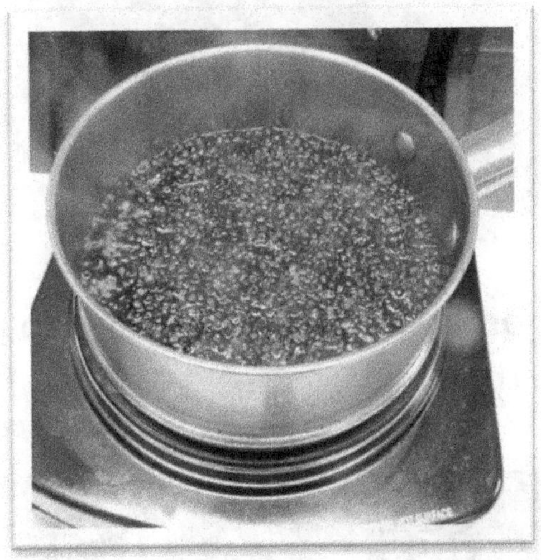

Strain using a coffee filter, jelly bag or muslin cloth.

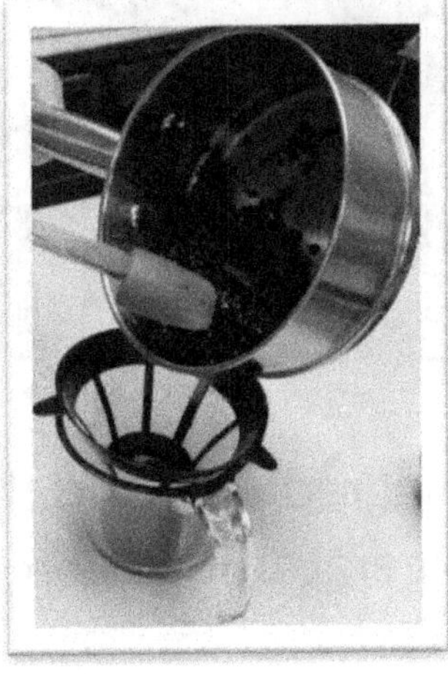

Measure the amount of tea and add equal amount of honey to taste and the lemon juice.

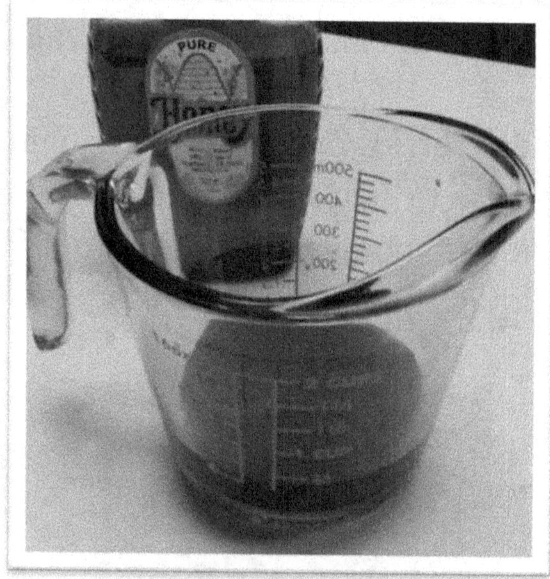

Pour into dark bottles or jars. It is much easier to pour up a teaspoon or syrup from a bottle than a jar.

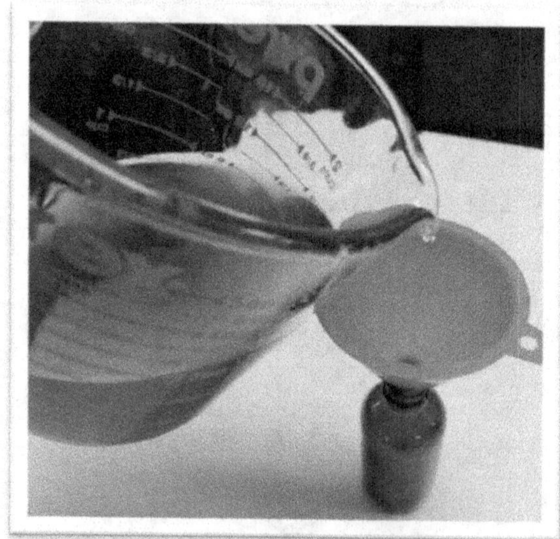

Label with the name of the ingredients and the date.
This should keep in the refrigerator for 1-2 months.

Optional: Pour into several small jars, leaving enough head room and freeze for a longer shelf life.

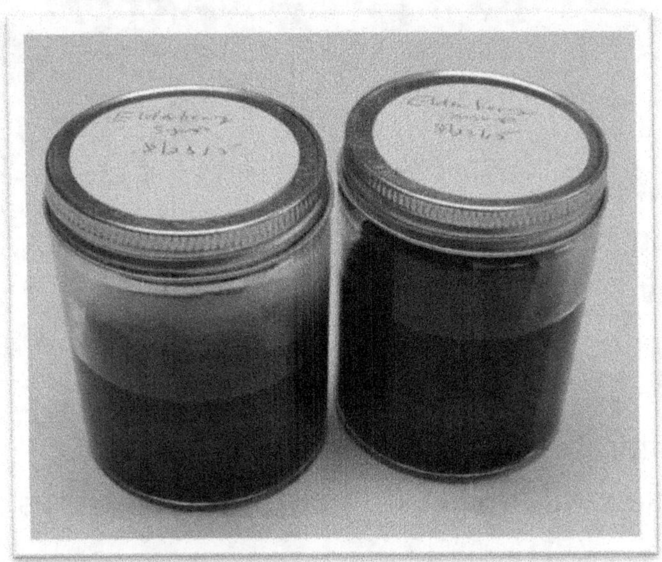

Elderberry Syrup, Even Longer Shelf Life
Add an equal amount of herbal tincture (this could be Echinacea or even an elderberry tincture) or Everclear. This would be 1 part herbal tea, 1 part honey and 1 part of Herbal tincture or Everclear.

Use the same ingredients except the lemon juice to make an herb infused honey.

ONION HONEY SYRUP
FOR COUGHS

1 large Onion
Deep Bowl
Honey

Slice a large onion into slices and place into a deep bowl.
Cover with honey.
Let stand overnight.
Strain.
Store in the refrigerator
Take a spoonful several times throughout the day or as needed.

GARLIC HONEY SYRUP TO BREAK UP CONGESTION

½ cup of finely minced garlic
½ cup of honey

Finely minced cloves of garlic. Let sit 10-15 minutes. The garlic cells
must be ruptured to release two separate chemicals of the garlic, alliin
and alliinase which then form a new compound called allicin.

Place the garlic in an 8 oz. jar.
Put in half of the honey.
Stir well.
Add rest of the honey.
Stir again.
 Add more honey if necessary to go to the top of the jar and put a lid
on.

Let sit in the refrigerator or on the counter top overnight.
No need to strain.

Store in the refrigerator.

How to Make Oxymels

Oxymels are basically your herb of choice, vinegar and honey. Oxymels will keep for many months, for longer storage, keep in the refrigerator. Take by the spoonful or add to hot water to drink as a hot tea.

Ginger Oxymel

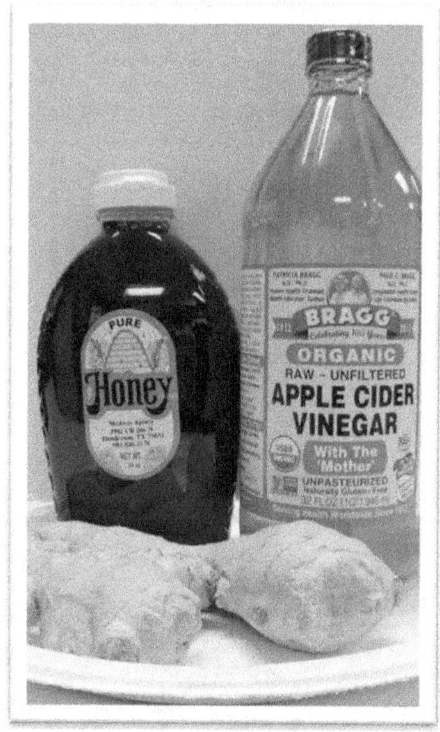

Take as an immune builder and to help thin mucus.
Ginger is a mild anti-inflammatory. Adding the optional Turmeric will boost this effect.
Ginger helps ease nausea and vomiting.
Ginger is the number one choice for motion sickness and is as effective as Dramamine and will not make you sleepy.

Oxymels

Fill any size jar 1/3 to ½ full of chopped or minced herb. Use the lesser amount if using dried herbs.

Fill the jar 2/3 full with apple cider vinegar.

Fill the jar to the top with honey.

Cap and label the jar with the name of the ingredients and the date.

Shake 2x a day for 2-6 weeks.

Add more honey and vinegar if necessary to keep herbs covered.

Strain and label.

1. Fill a jar 1/3 full of grated fresh ginger. Optional: Add 1 tablespoon of dried turmeric.

2. Fill the jar 2/3 full of apple cider vinegar.

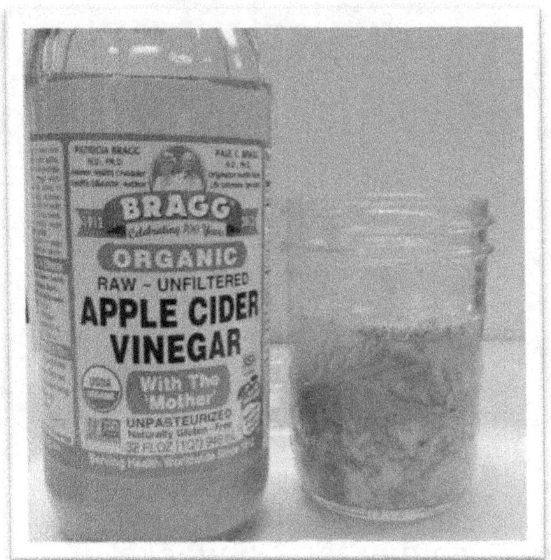

3. Fill the jar to the top with honey.

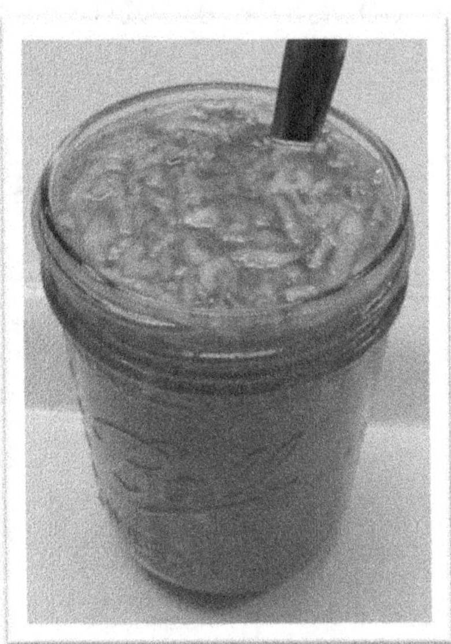

4. Stir the herb, vinegar and honey mixture.

5. Cap and label with the name of the herbs, solvent (vinegar and honey), and date.

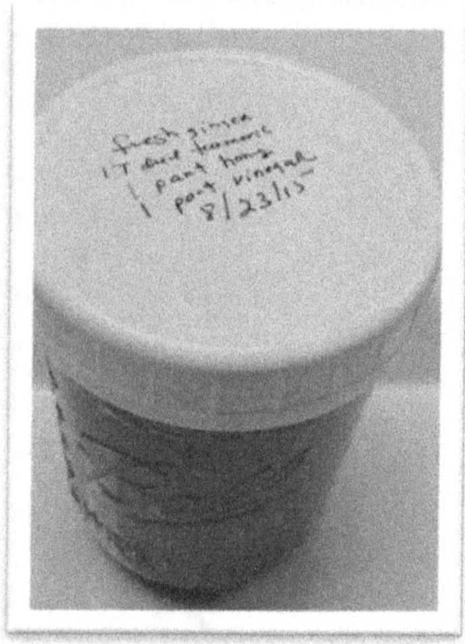

6. Shake each day for 2-6 weeks.
You may need to add more vinegar and honey if the herbs do not remain covered.

7. Strain and pour into a bottle or jar.

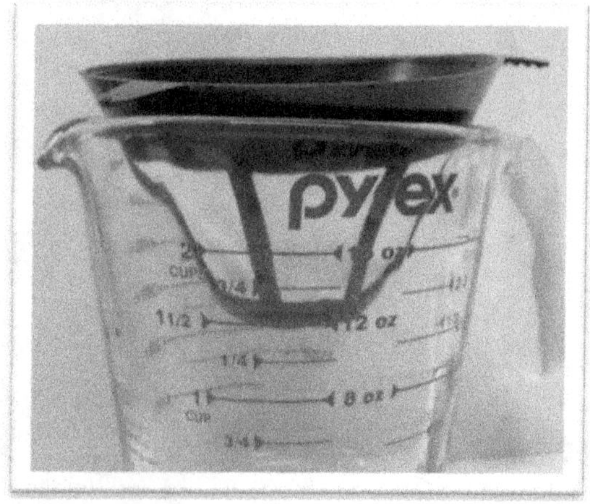

8. Label with the name of the Oxymel and the date.

Oxymels can also be used as the base for a marinade or dressing by adding olive oil to it.
Turn any herbal vinegar into an oxymel by adding honey to it.

Tips on peeling and grating ginger.

Use a spoon to peel ginger.

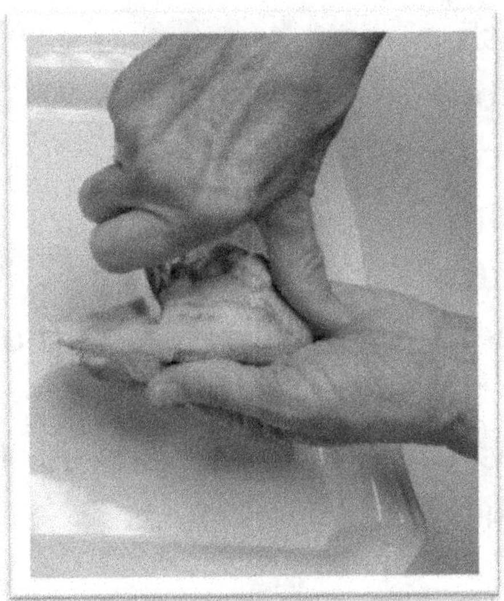

Caution: Ginger may cause heartburn or be too spicy for some.

GARLIC CIDER VINEGAR

There are many variations of this recipe. The main ingredients are the cloves of garlic, peppers and apple cider vinegar. If you are using horseradish the cooler months are the only time fresh horseradish is available. Anti viral herbs are then added. Use what you have, do not let the lack of the other ingredients keep you from making Garlic Cider Vinegar.

10 cloves of garlic, minced let set 10-15 minutes.
½ cup grated or chopped ginger
½ cup grated horseradish
1 medium chopped onion
2 chopped jalapeno or cayenne peppers
Zest and juice of 1 lemon
Several sprigs of rosemary
1 tablespoon of powdered turmeric or 1/4 cup of fresh grated turmeric root
Optional spices such as cinnamon and cloves. (The spice Clove buds, not more cloves of Garlic.

Combine in a quart jar. Some recipes say heat the vinegar, others say do not. If you are using regular store bought pasteurized vinegar, there are no living enzymes to kill. If you are using unpasteurized organic apple cider vinegar with the mother do not heat so as not to kill the enzymes. Heat apple cider vinegar until warm, do not boil or over heat, you do not want to kill the enzymes. Add the apple cider vinegar to the jar and cover with a plastic lid. If you only have a metal lid place a piece of plastic wrap between the lid and the jar to prevent the vinegar from corroding the lid.

Store in a cool dark place for 1 month, shaking daily. Strain and then add 1/4 cup of honey or to taste.

This should be good for a couple of months sitting out. Store this in the refrigerator for longer storage.

Take a spoonful at a time at the first sign of a cold or continue to take once you become sick. I add it to hot water to drink as a hot tea when I have congestion or other symptoms of cold or allergies.

This can also be used to make oil and vinegar dressing or vegetable marinades.

Garlic Cider Vinegar Dressing or Marinade
1/4 cup of Garlic Cider Vinegar
1/4 cup olive oil
2 tablespoons of spicy southwest ground mustard or other mustard of your choice. Mustard not only adds flavor but also acts as an emulsifier.

GARLIC & HONEY FOR INFECTIONS

Garlic is considered nature's antibiotic. Of course most know that a cold or flu is not a bacterium so it will not respond to antibiotics. Garlic like most herbs are not an antibiotic, they are antimicrobial which means virus, fungus or bacteria.

When using garlic as an antibiotic or antimicrobial, the garlic must be raw. Mince the garlic and let it set 10-15 minutes. The garlic cells must be ruptured to release two separate chemicals of the garlic, alliin and alliinase which then form a new compound called allicin.

Eating too much garlic at once may cause tummy problems, so start slowly and build up.

1. Mince 3-5 cloves of garlic. Let set 10-15 minutes.

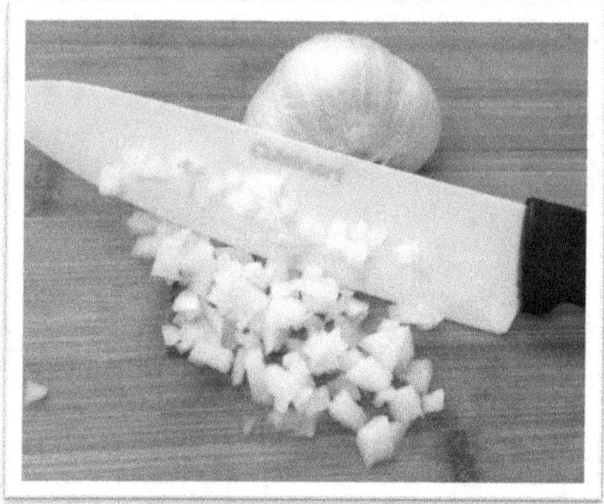

2. Place 1 tablespoon of honey on a plate.
Optional: Add 1/8 teaspoon or a pinch of powdered cayenne pepper.
Add the minced garlic and mix together.
Take a spoonful once an hour or at least 3-4 times a day.

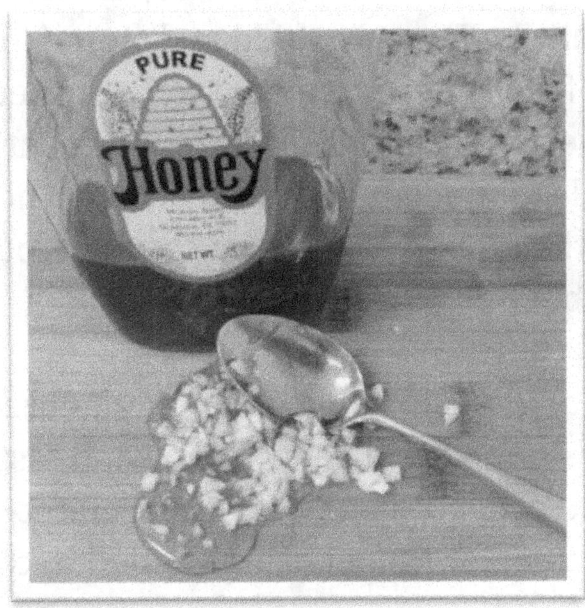

3. The honey will stick to the throat, the cayenne pepper will increase circulation and the garlic will stimulate the immune system.

SLIPPERY ELM THROAT AND TUMMY SOOTHERS

Although many herbalists will call these lozenges I do not because the first thing one thinks of is the hard candy cough drops. The hard candy type cough drops are brought to a hard boil, which would destroy the benefits of honey. These throat soothers are formed from dried powdered herbs, Licorice Root tea and honey and some have the addition of essential oils. They are dried and stored in the refrigerator for the longest shelf life. They are meant to be sucked on so that the mucilage will soothe and moisten your throat by coating it. If they were not dried they would immediately dissolve in your mouth and then they wouldn't be doing their job. A few can be carried around in a tin in your purse or pocket to be used as needed.

Marshmallow root or Plantain could be used but I prefer the Slippery Elm. Marshmallow Root has a distinct aroma and taste which I suppose some herbalists just love, but I guess it is an acquired taste that I have not acquired. Cinnamon or Ginger can be added to the Slippery Elm Powder.

Other herbal teas can be used instead of Licorice Root tea. Licorice Root adds that extra sweetness along with a flavor many are familiar with. It has antiviral properties and is a demulcent.
These recipes are a base from which you can get started with and then create and adjust for your own individual taste and needs.

Slippery Elm Throat Soothers begin with a strong Licorice Root Tea.

Strong Licorice Tea
1 teaspoon of chopped Licorice Root or ½ teaspoon of powder
½ cup of water

Combine the water and the Licorice Root and simmer in a covered pan for 10-15 minutes or until the tea is reduced to ¼ cup.

If you do not have or cannot find Licorice Root, you could use any of the herbal teas with Licorice Root as the main ingredient such as:
Traditional Medicinals: Throat Coat
Stash: Licorice Spice
Both of these are available at Drug Emporium and health food stores.

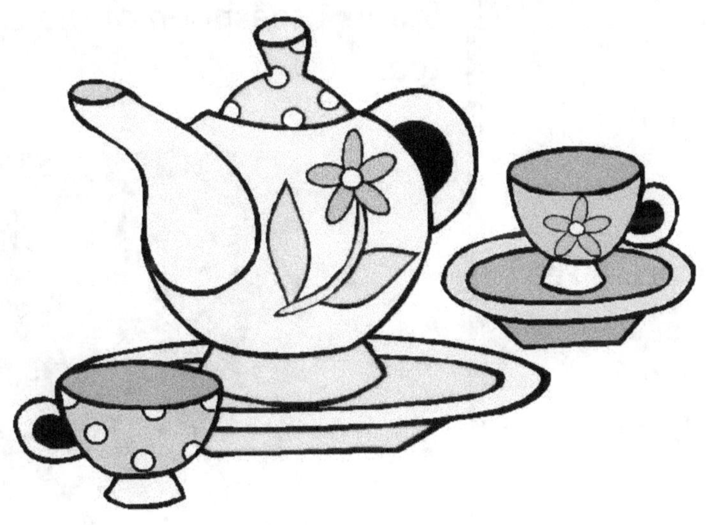

Slippery Elm Throat Soothers

Slipper Elm Throat Soothers

4 teaspoon of strong Licorice Root Tea

2 tablespoons of Slippery Elm Powder plus extra for rolling

1 tablespoon of honey

Strong Licorice Tea

1 teaspoon of chopped Licorice Root
Or ½ teaspoon powder

½ cup of water

4 teaspoons of strong Licorice Root tea
2 tablespoons of Slippery Elm powder plus extra for rolling
1 tablespoon of honey
Small bowl or plate
Upside down paper plate
Wax or parchment paper
Rolling pin

1. Place 1 tablespoon of Slippery Elm Powder in a small bowl or small plate. Stir in 1 teaspoon of the Licorice Root tea.

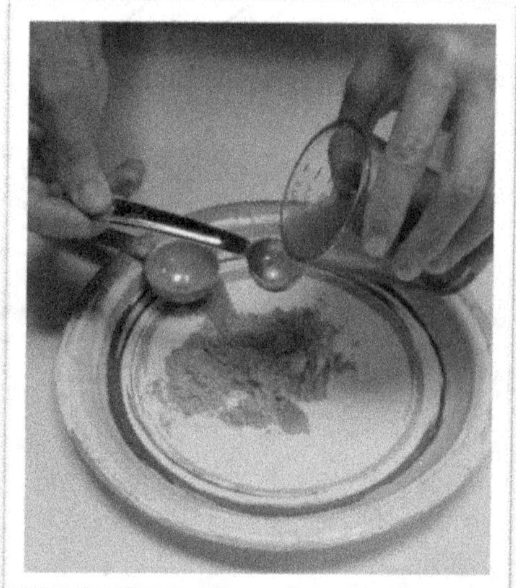

2. Continue to stir in the remaining 3 teaspoons of Licorice Root Tea 1 teaspoon at a time until thoroughly moistened.

3. Stir in 1 tablespoon of honey.

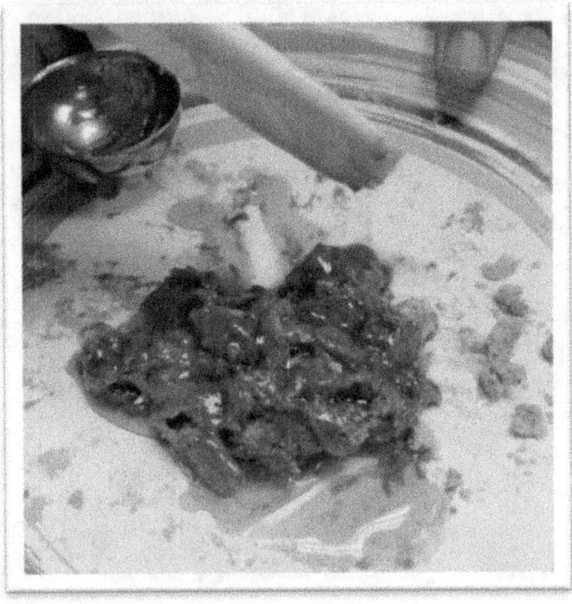

4. Lay down wax or parchment paper.
Place 1 tablespoon of Slippery Elm powder on the paper.
Pour honey mixture over the Slippery Elm powder.

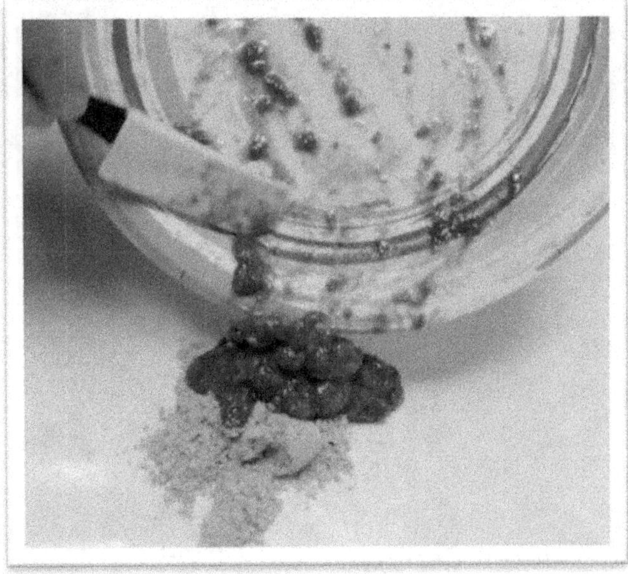

5. Mix all ingredients together.

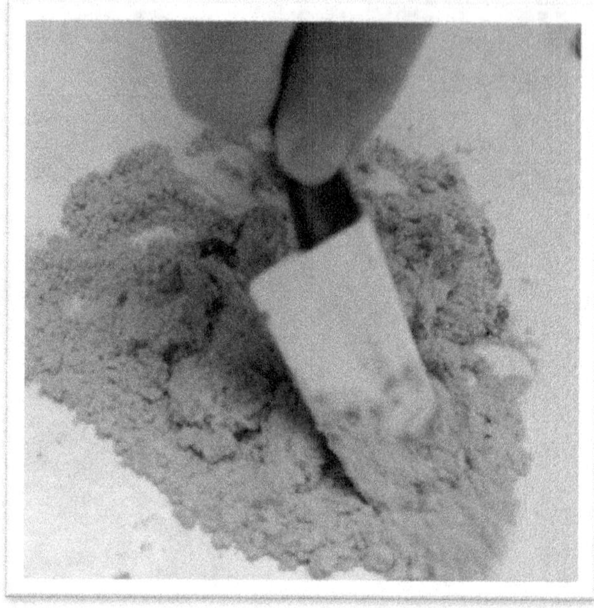

6. Continue to mix the mixture with your hands, forming into a ball like you would a pie crust.

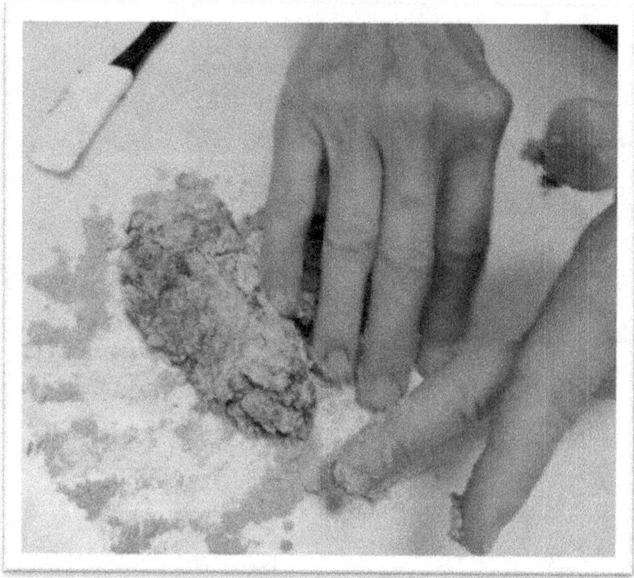

7. Sprinkle the additional Slippery Elm powder onto the wax or parchment paper and dust the rolling pin with the Slippery Elm powder.

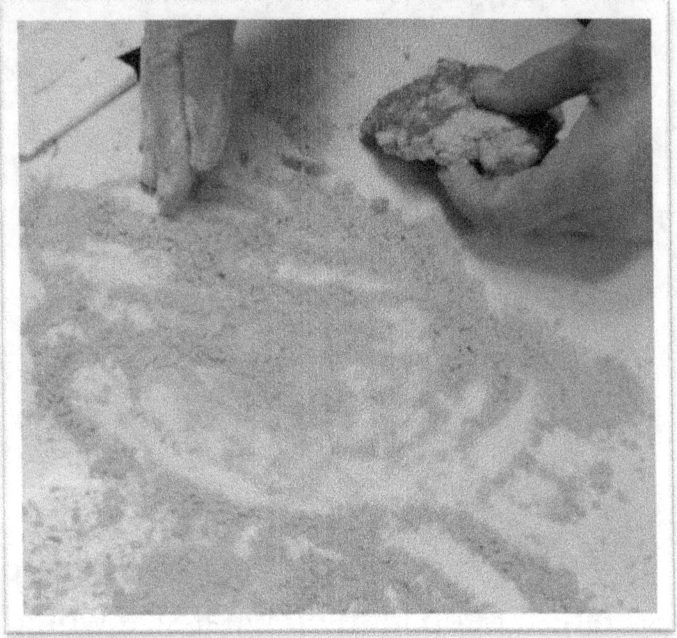

8. Roll out to about ¼ inch thick. Add more Slippery Elm powder if needed.

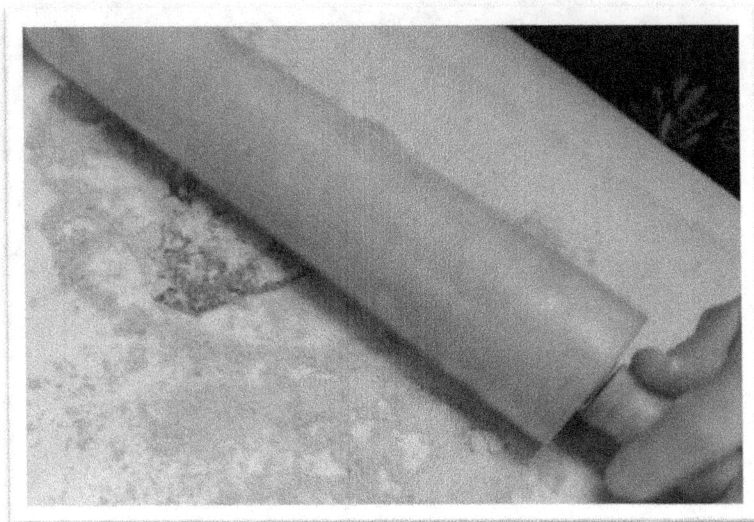

9. Use a bottle cap to cut out small circles.

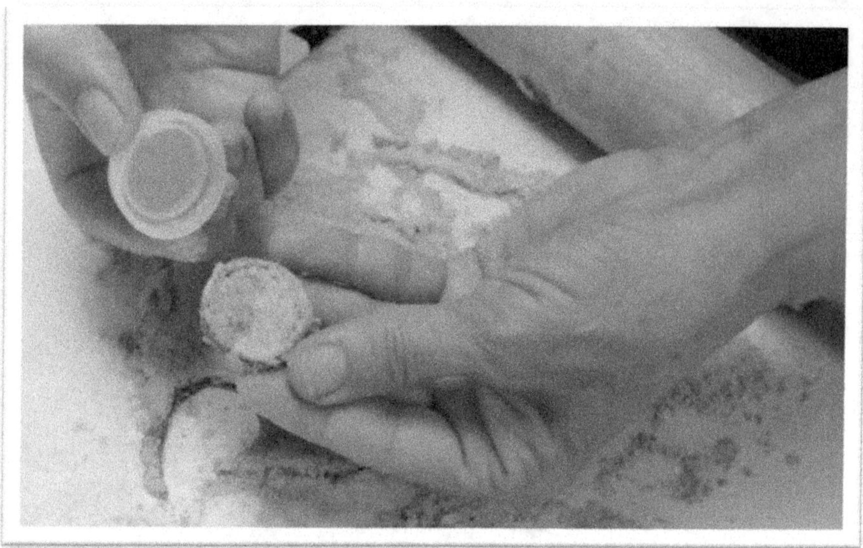

Or if you do not have that kind of patience, use a knife or a pizza cutter to cut into small squares. Keep in mind what size would be comfortable in your mouth.

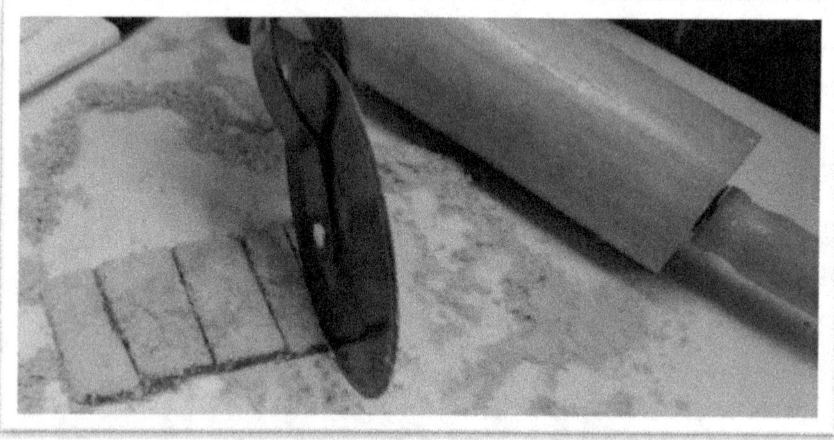

10. Dry on top of a paper plate turned upside down. Turn each day until completely dry. A dehydrator or an oven with a light bulb could be used.

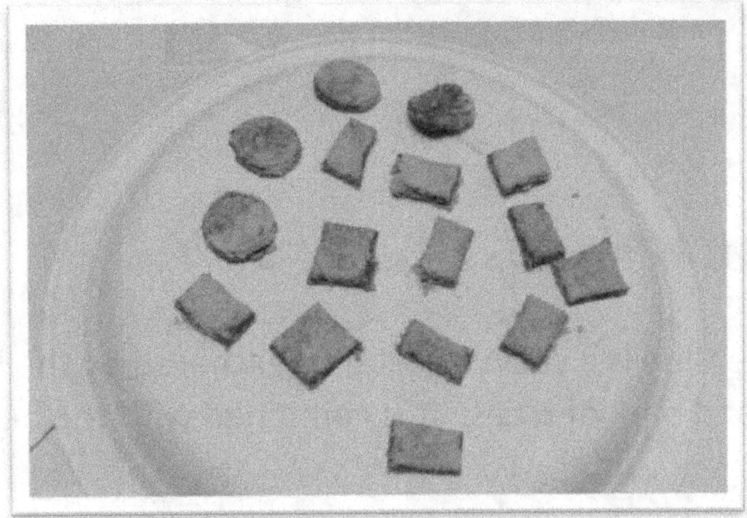

They are not pretty to look at and are dry when you first put them in your mouth. They are very soothing to the throat once you start to suck on them.

I had one student tell me they helped with her dry mouth.

4 Healing with Propolis

Propolis or Bee Glue is a sticky substance gathered by the bees from the leaf buds and bark of trees. It is combined with the bees' secretions.

It is used in the hives to seal holes and cracks, protect the hives from cold and rain, and used and act as an antibacterial and antifungal protecting the hives from disease and infections.

Bee propolis has been used since ancient times for healing wounds, ulcers, sores and soothes inflammation.
In the 17th century, propolis was listed as an official drug in the London pharmacopoeias.

As with other bee products, if you are allergic to bees you could have an allergy to propolis. As a precaution try a small amount for the first time to see how you react to it.

 Propolis can be powdered and taken in capsule form or added to honey or other preparations. I have not had much luck powdering propolis. It is sold in health food stores and on the internet if you wish to try it. Another bee keeper told me that she will swallow a small amount of propolis and it makes her feel great.

Propolis must first be made into a tincture or an oil before it can be used in the recipes and remedies I have provided in this book, such as lotions and salves.

You can take the propolis tincture or the oil orally.

When cleaning up propolis, use any kind of vegetable or nut oil. Alcohol, water or any kind of soap will not clean up propolis. Be prepared to throw away your containers used to make propolis tincture. The propolis oil will clean up with oil, and then washed with soap and hot water.

Tinctures of propolis and propolis oil can be used to treat burns, wounds, all kinds of skin conditions, used for mouth sores, and used as a mouthwash. It not only heals wounds faster but helps stimulate new tissue growth.

Keep in mind applying propolis tincture, being alcohol will burn open wounds and burns. You might find the propolis oil is better.

From our experience the tincture of propolis is very effective relieving bee and wasp stings.

Respiratory infections respond to propolis when combined with Vitamin C.

Propolis is very effective applied topically to both prevent infections and treat infections of wounds and burns. It is not as effective internally.

A study comparing Brazilian propolis cream to a silver sulfadiazine salve treating minor burns showed those using the propolis cream showed less inflammation and more rapid closure. There was no difference in microbial growth.

Propolis is effective against gram positive bacteria such as:
Staphylococcus: causes wound and urinary tract infections
Clostridium: causes gastrointestinal distress
Corynebacterium diptheriae: causes diphtheria
Some strains of Streptococcus: causes strep throat, sinus infections, and scarlet fever
Klebsiella pneumonia: causes pneumonia and bronchitis
Pseudomonas: causes wound infections

It does not work as well with gram negative bacteria such as:
Escherichia coli, Shigella: causes dysentery
Salmonella: causes gastrointestinal distress.

So you can see all illness is not caused by the same bacteria. So propolis may or may not work for you depending on which bacteria are causing the problem.

Propolis as a mouthwash:
I normally squirt a dropper full of propolis tincture in a little water to use as a mouthwash.
Propolis as a mouthwash is effective against common oral bacteria that may cause bad breath, periodontal disease such as gingivitis and periodontitis, tooth decay and prevent plaque build- up.

Anti-fungal properties:
Propolis is shown to be effective against:
 Microsporum which cause ringworm and a tropical skin and scalp fungal disease
Trichtophyton: which causes skin and nail infections.
Note: Propolis is not effective if the disease is deeply embedded in the skin or is internal.
Candida: common yeast infection

Anti-viral:
Effective against cold virus and herpes simplex virus including cold sores and genital herpes.

Properties of propolis:
More than 180 phytochemicals including flavonoids (potent anti-oxidants), organic acids and their derivatives: anti-fungal, phytosterols, and essential oil compounds. These compounds are known to have biological activities such as anti-inflammatory, anti-microbial, antimutagentic, antihistamine, and anti-allergenic properties.

Propolis Tincture 10% Strength

Weigh 1 part propolis

Weigh 9 parts vodka or other alcohol 75 proof or higher

Mix together in a glass container with a tight fitting lid.

Store in a dark place for 1-2 weeks.
Shake daily 2-3 times.

Strain and keep in a dark container.

Propolis is about 30% beeswax. All of it will not dissolve.

How to Make Propolis Tincture 10% Strength

1. Weigh 1 part propolis
2. Weigh 9 parts alcohol

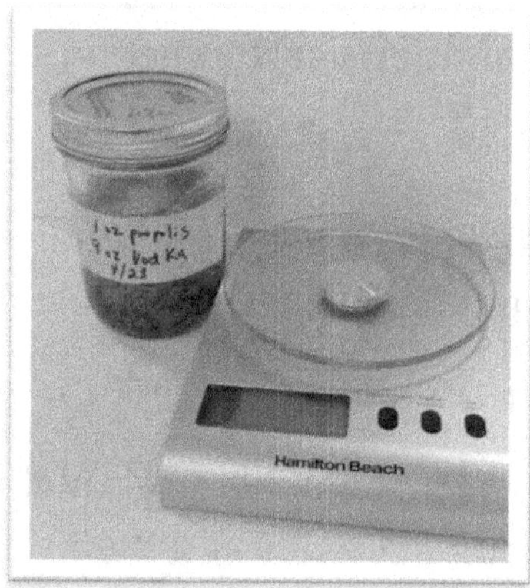

3. Mix together in a glass container with a tight fitting lid. Label with the name of the ingredients and date.

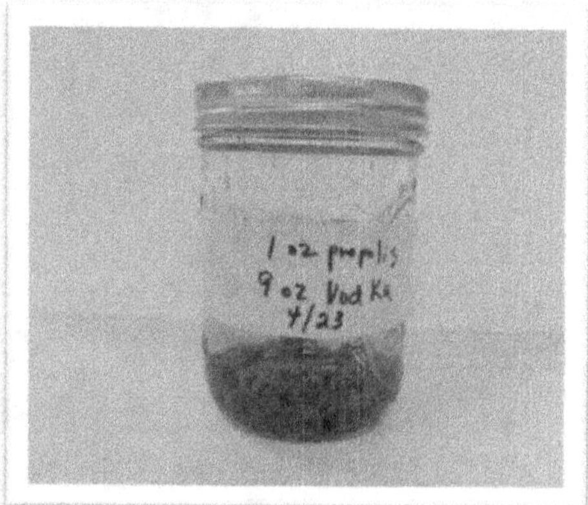

4. Store in a dark place. Shake 2-3 times daily for 1-2 weeks.
Storing in a dark place can be as simple as placing a towel over the jar.
If I stored my tincture in a dark place I would forget about it.

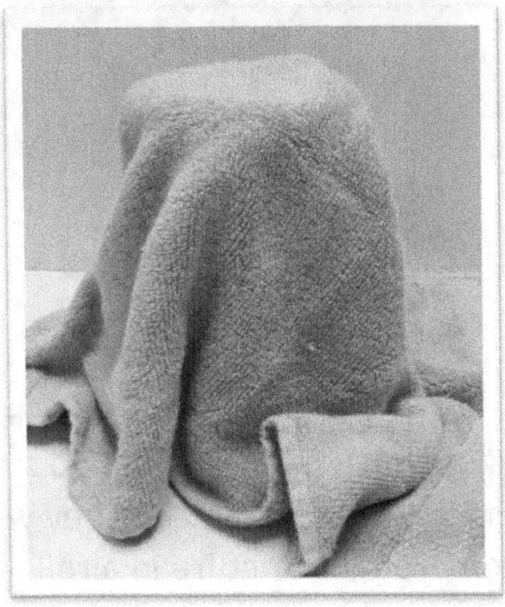

5. Strain using a re-useable coffee filter, layered cheesecloth, paper coffee filters, or muslin.
If the tincture is not strained fine enough you will get tiny bits of propolis and beeswax stuck to your teeth when you take it by mouth, use it as a mouthwash or a gargle.

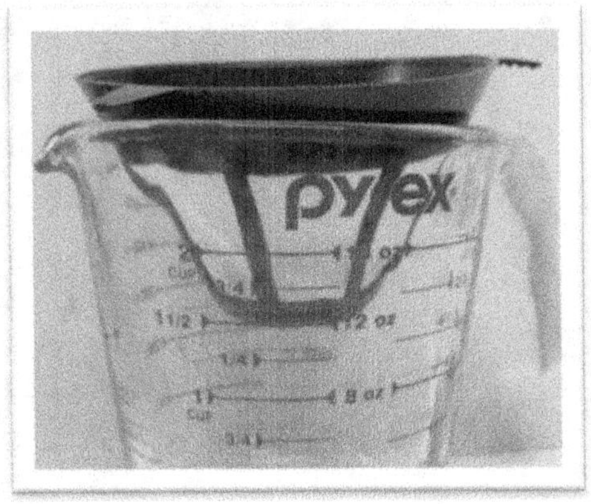

6. Pour into a dark colored bottle.

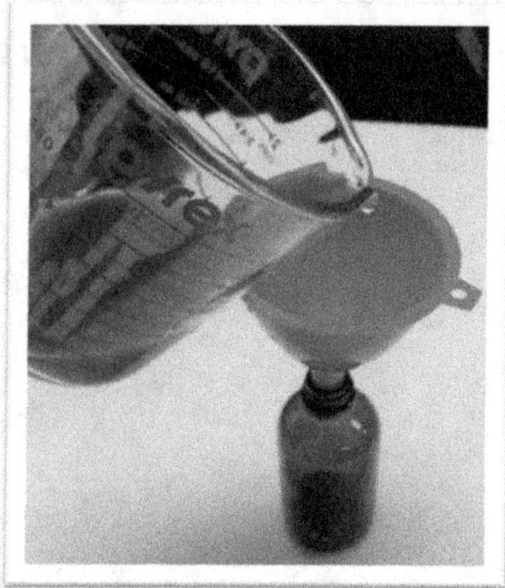

You can store in one large bottle and then fill up small bottles as you need them. As you use the propolis bottles they will become sticky and glue the lid shut. I keep propolis tincture in a roll –on- bottle for bee and wasp stings. The dark colored roll- on- bottle is the best but is more expensive. If the clear roll on bottle is all that you can find that is ok also.

I keep some in a spray bottle for spraying my throat, mouth, wounds, etc.

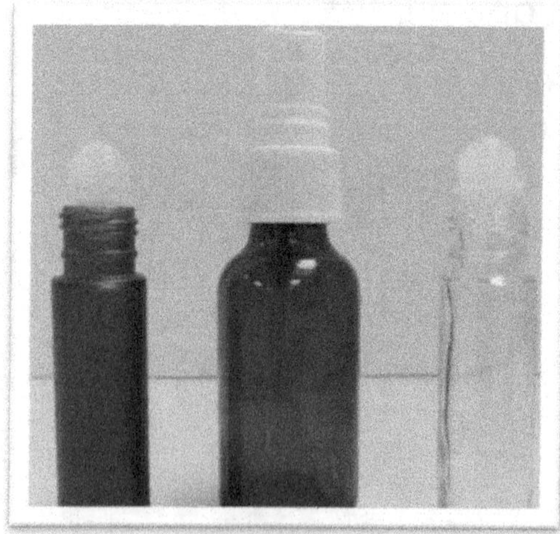

Propolis Infused Oil

10 grams of propolis by weight (about 1 tablespoon)

200 ml of olive oil or other oil, measured (about 6.7 oz.)

Heat keeping under 122 ◦f for 10 minutes or more.

Or, heat in a yogurt maker overnight keeping it around 100◦f or

No Heat Method
Mix in a sealed container and store for 2 weeks in the dark.
Shake 2-3 times a day. Strain into a dark colored bottle.

How to Make Propolis Infused Oil

1. Weigh 10 grams of propolis.

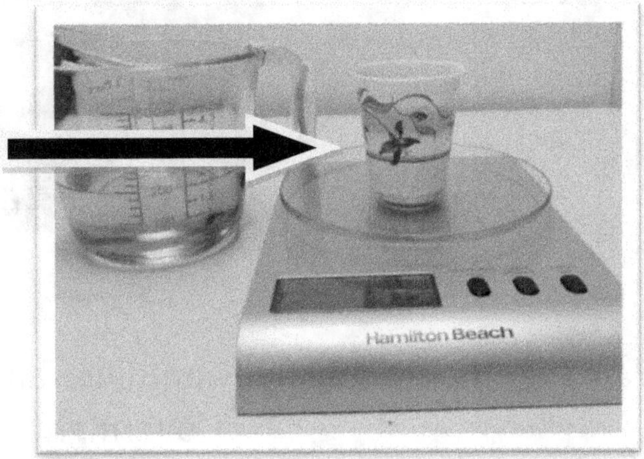

2. Measure 200 ml of olive oil or other oil.

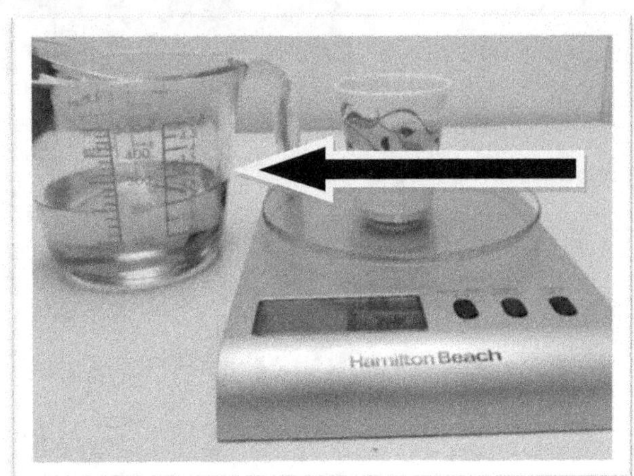

3. Heat in a double boiler for 10 minutes or more.
Use a thermometer to make sure the temperature stays below 122°f.

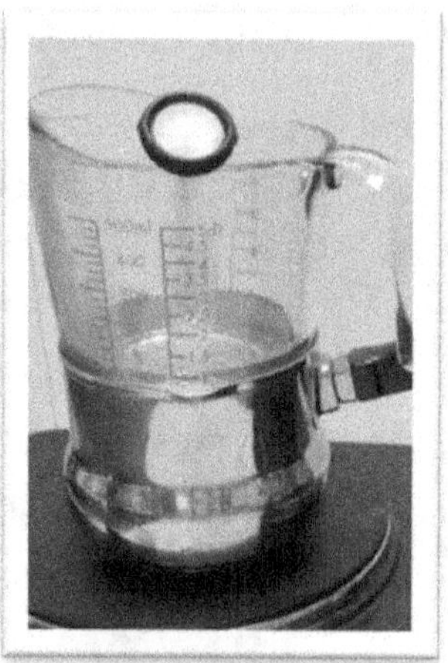

Or
Mix together in a sealed container and place in a yogurt maker
overnight.

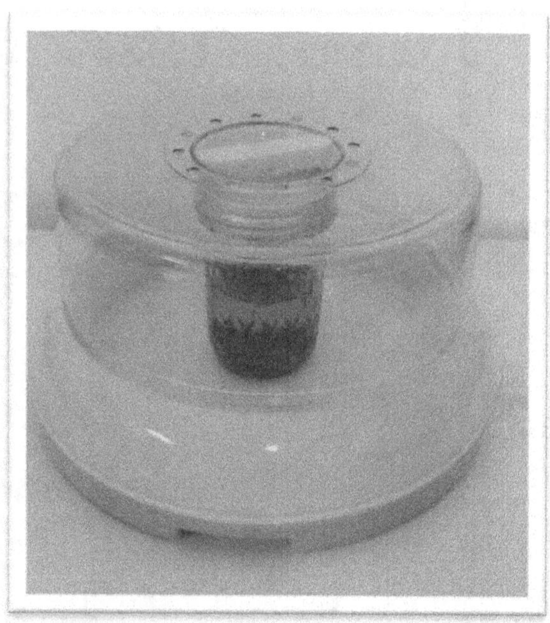

Notice the lid does not close all the way on the yogurt maker. Monitor
the temperature so it does not go over 122°f.

Or, No Heat Method

Mix in a sealed jar.

Label your jar with the ingredients and the date.

Store in a dark place for 2 weeks.

Shake 2-3 times a day.

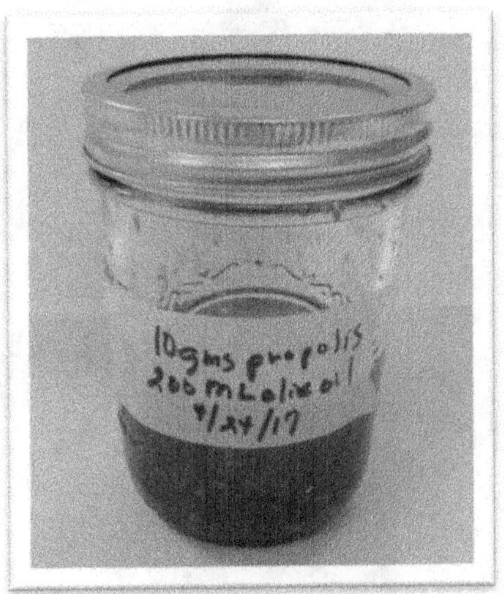

Strain: Use a re-useable coffee filter, cheesecloth or a paper filter. If you do not strain fine enough you will have bits of propolis and beeswax left wherever it is applied.

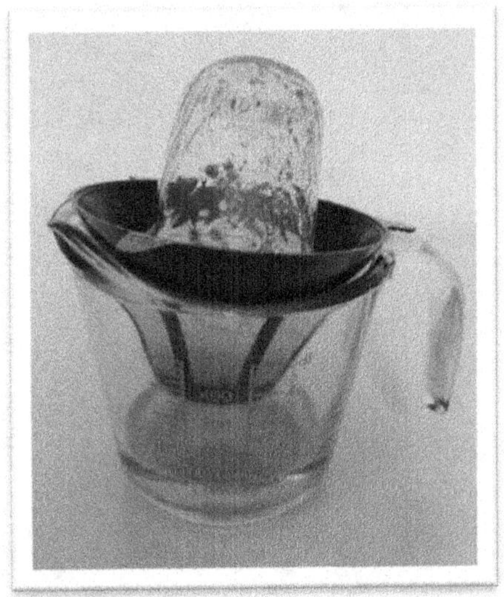

Store in a dark colored bottle.
Label the bottle with the ingredients and the date.

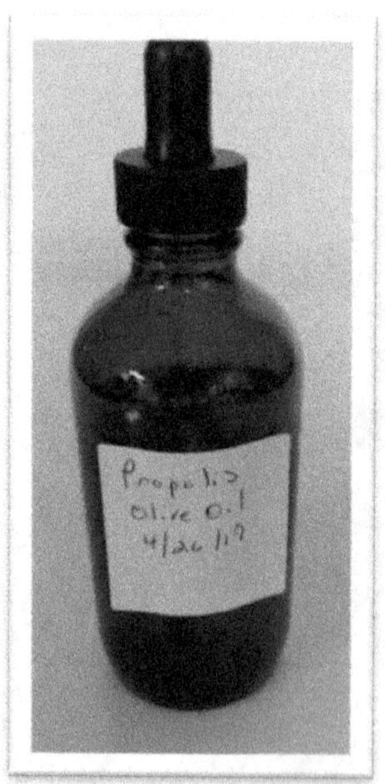

You are now ready to make salves and lotions with propolis oil.
Unlike Propolis Tincture, propolis oil will clean up from you equipment
and containers that were used.

HEALING PROPOLIS SALVE, OINTMENT OR BALM

Ointments, salves and balms are all the same thing, oil thickened with beeswax or other wax.

Put it into a small tube and it becomes a lip balm, a larger tube and it is a cuticle balm, a heel balm or whatever balm you wish it to be.

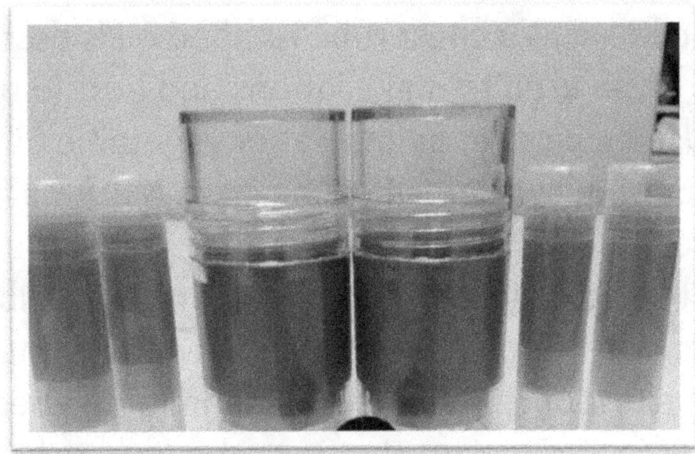

Pour it into a jar or a larger container and it is now an ointment.

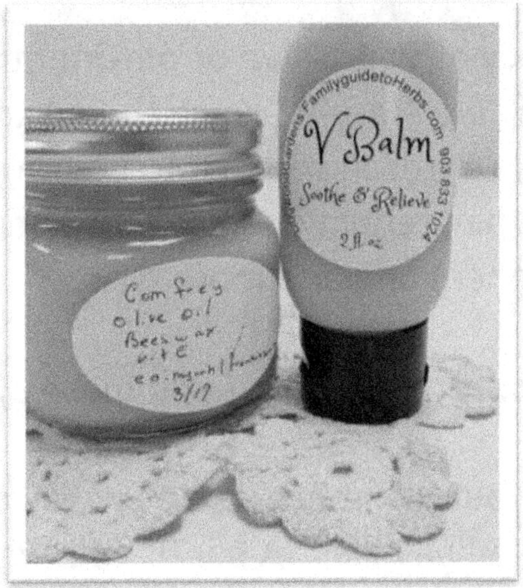

A propolis ointment or salve begins with propolis infused oil. The propolis oil is then thickened with beeswax. Approximately, 1 oz. (about 4 tablespoons) of beeswax per 8 oz. of propolis oil. Adding essential oils are optional.

Most medical infused oils are made with a base of olive oil. Castor oil has its own healing benefits and makes very thick oil.   Castor oil would be especially beneficial as a chest rub. Almond oil is best for the lips. Grapeseed oil is often used to make lotions and best for the face.
 Our ancestors used whatever animal fat or vegetable oil that they had. Although coconut oil is awesome healing oil, it is normally combined with other oils to offset its property of turning into a liquid or solid state at various temperatures.   There are countless recipes and methods using various combinations of oils. Making smaller amounts and using the smallest of containers is recommended because the ointment or salve can go rancid. The first time you stick your finger into a jar of salve or ointment, you have contaminated it, another reason to use the smallest of containers.

Testing the consistency of your salve or ointment:
Place metal spoons in your freezer. Once the oil and beeswax is completely melted, dip a frozen spoon into your mixture.
If your remedy is too thin, reheat and use more beeswax. If you remedy is too hard, reheat and add more oil.

Not enough infused propolis oil? Just add more of another oil.

Unless you are using your own beeswax, beeswax comes in bars or beads, sometimes called pastilles. A bar of beeswax is almost impossible to melt and measure. I prefer the beeswax beads.

Propolis Salve, Balm or Ointment

Large Recipe:
8 oz. of propolis oil by measurement

1 oz. of beeswax by weight. (2 oz. if making tubes)

Optional: 12-20 drops of essential oil **per 1 oz. of oil**

Makes 1-8 oz. container
Or 2-4 oz. container
Or 4 -2 oz. container.

Propolis Salve, Balm or Ointment Large Recipe

1. Measure 8 oz. of propolis infused oil.

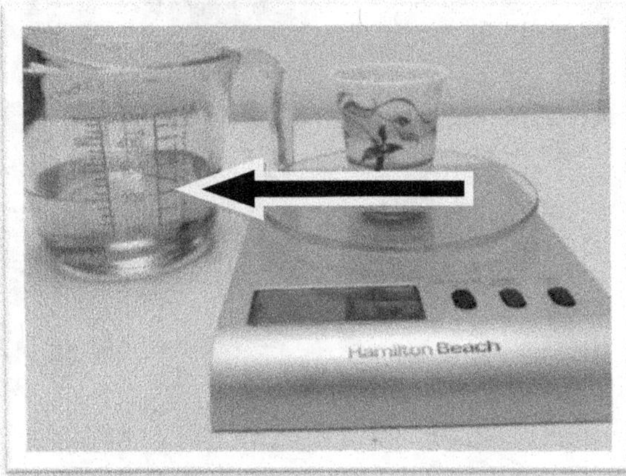

2. Weigh 1 oz. of beeswax. (About 4 tablespoons if you do not have a scale.)

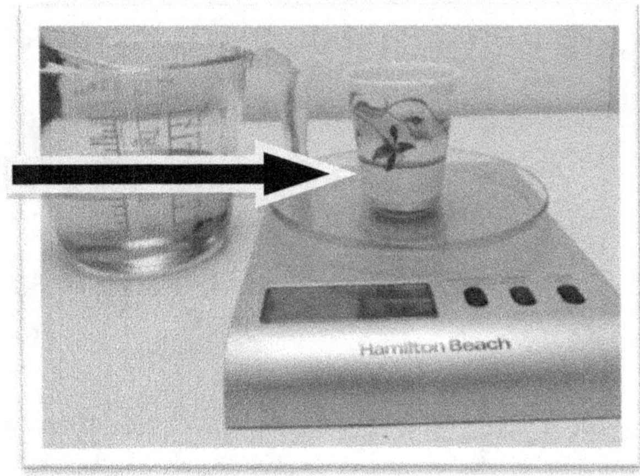

3. Place a towel next to your double boiler and have your containers ready. You need the towel to wipe off the bottom of the pan to prevent dripping water into your salve. I slide the pan on the towel to remove the water. Have plenty of paper towels nearby.

4. Melt the beeswax in the top of the double boiler.

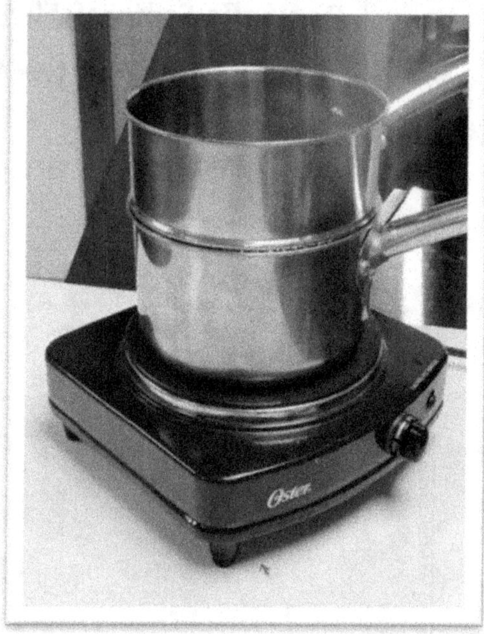

5. Stir in the Propolis Oil into the melted beeswax.
Melting the beeswax first limits the Propolis Oil's benefits being destroyed by the heat.

6. Remove from heat and place the pan on top of the towel.

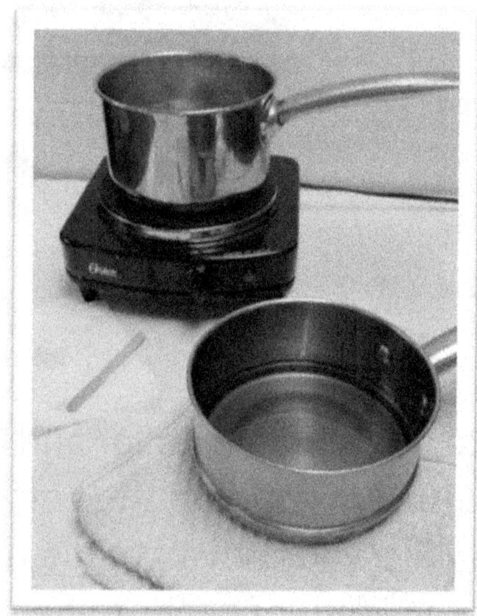

Pour into individual containers. When the bottom of the container starts to change colors, stir in the essential oils.

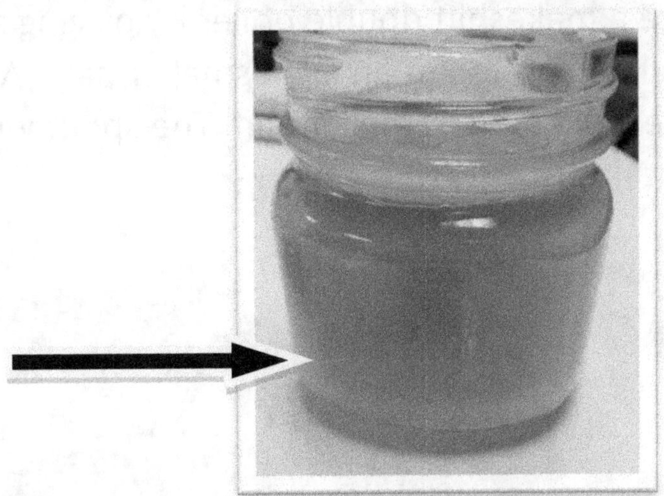

Do not cap until the salve has completely cooled. Placing the cap on the salve while still warm will cause condensation which may grow mold and bacteria.

Wipe container off with rubbing alcohol to remove any oil or wax. Apply label with name of ingredients and the date.

Making Smaller Recipes using Small Containers

When making smaller recipes you will want to use smaller heating utensils. You can make a makeshift double boiler by placing a measuring cup or small pan on top of an even smaller pan. A heatproof measuring glass can be placed on a smaller pan. The spout will be a plus pouring into small containers.

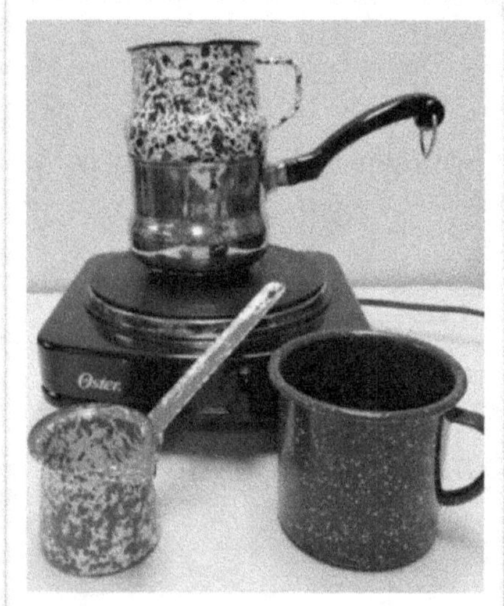
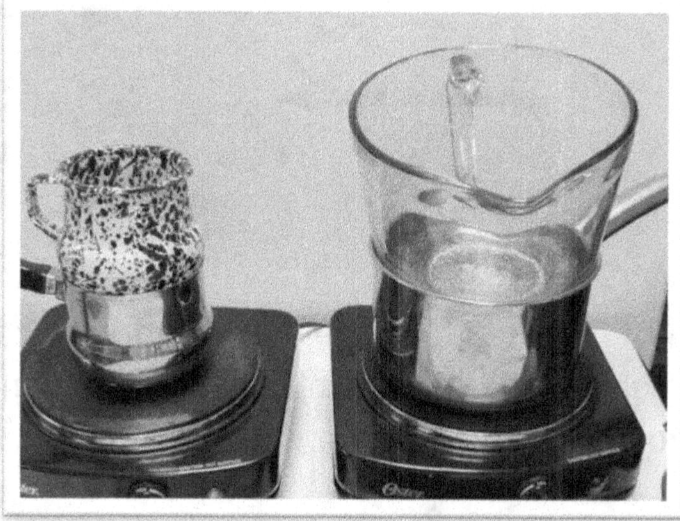

Remember to place the folded towel down to wipe the moisture off the bottom of the container. If you are really careful you can place a small pan directly on your burner. Do not place glass containers directly on the burner.

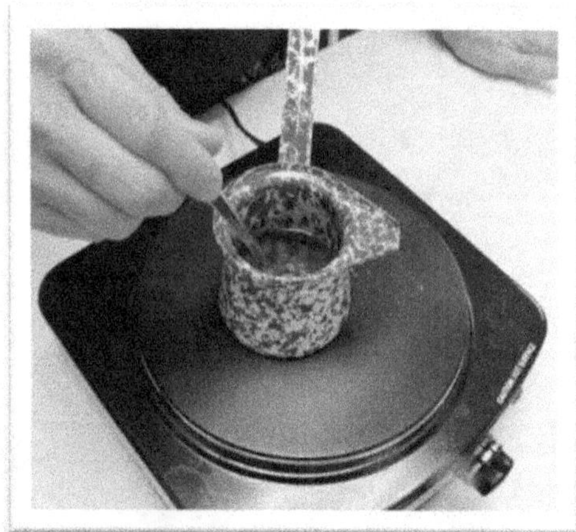

As your pour your lip balm out of the container, it will immediately start to harden on your container. You will need to set it back on your heat source to re-melt.

For cleaning purposes you can place glass containers in the microwave to re-melt and wipe out with a paper towel before washing.

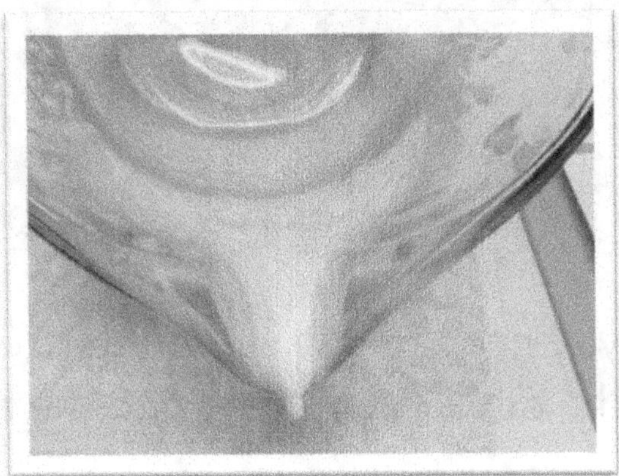

There are countless small containers you can use from small pots, tins and tubes.

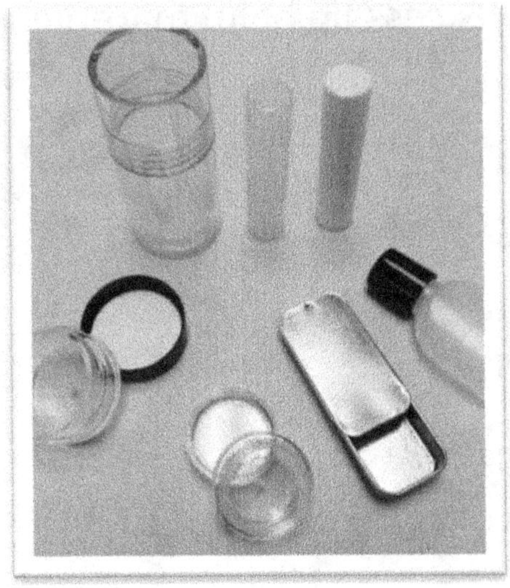

For small tubes you might want to invest in a filling tray.

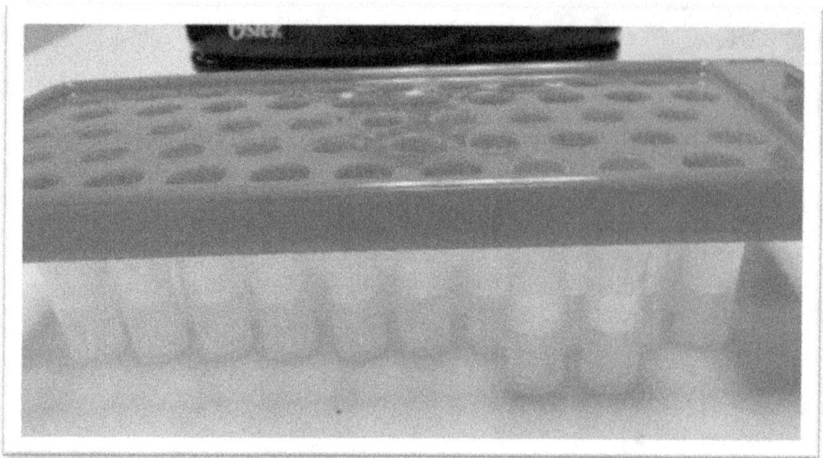

If using a filling tray, you need to buy your tubes from the same company to be sure the tubes fit properly into the trays.

When I first started making lip balm, I poured them individually into the tubes, which really takes a steady hand. Even though my customers loved them, I quit making them because it was too much to do. The filling trays make a big difference.

Notice the dimples and excess lip balm material.

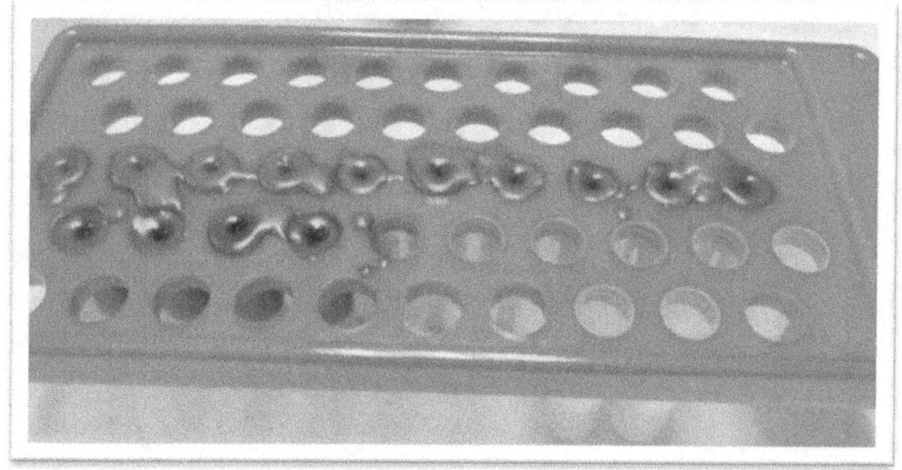

A scrapper will come with your filling tray. Use it to scrape off excess material to re-melt and fill in the holes.

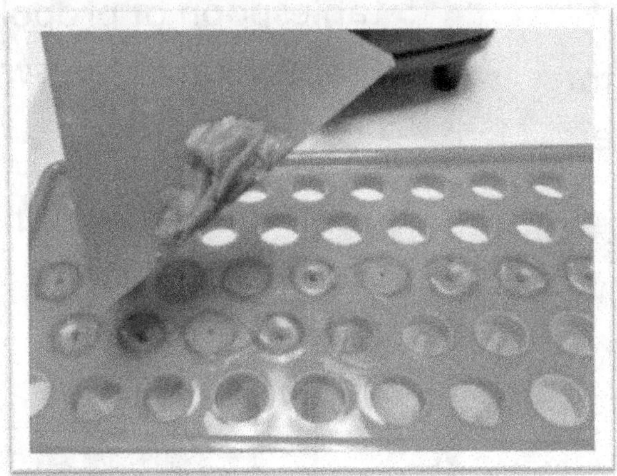

Or use a blow dryer to smooth out the lip balm material.

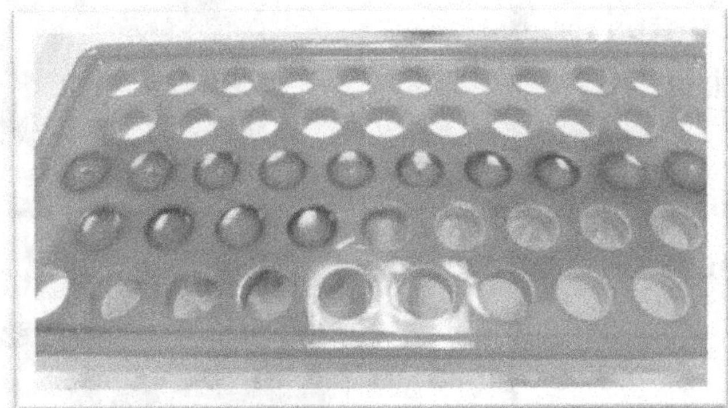

Adding essential oils to smaller recipes and smaller containers:
After removing your container from the heat, wait about 1 minute and then add your essential oils or flavorings. Depending on the room temperature and how your container retains the heat, you may even need to add your essential oils immediately after removing the container from its heat source. Only experience will tell you which you need to do.

Propolis Balm, Salve or Ointment

Small Recipe for small containers.

5 tablespoons of propolis oil

1 tablespoon of beeswax

Optional: up to 20 drops of essential oil or flavoring.

Makes about 20 - 3ml containers or 2 – ½ oz. containers.

Using Tubes:
5 tablespoons of propolis oil

2 tablespoons of beeswax

Propolis Balm, Salve or Ointment: Small Recipe

5 tablespoon of propolis oil
1 tablespoon of beeswax, 2 tablespoons if using tubes.

1. Melt the beeswax in a small double boiler or small pan.

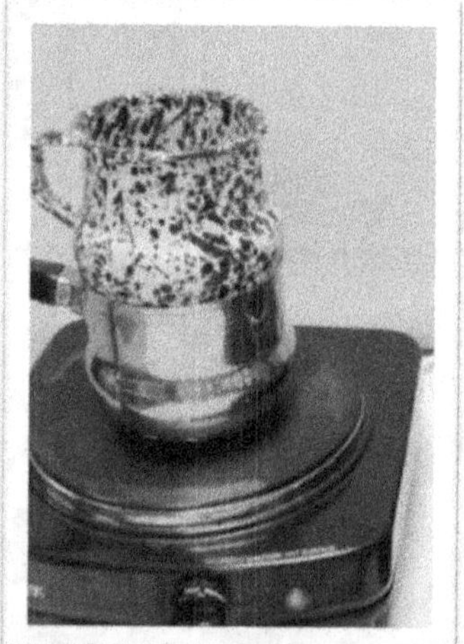

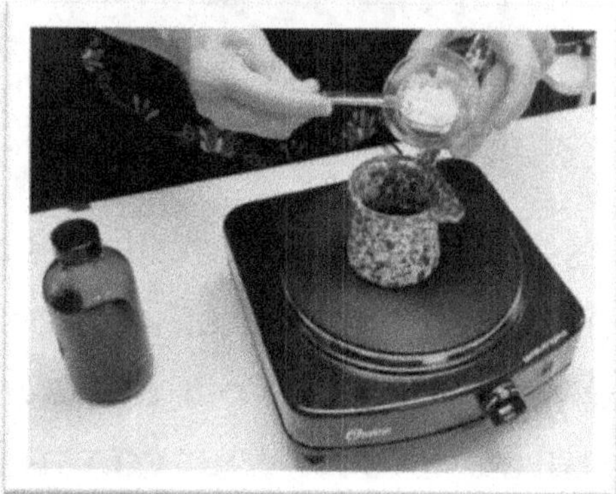

2. Stir the propolis oil into the melted beeswax. Melting the beeswax first limits the propolis oil's benefits being destroyed by heat.

3. Remove from heat. Placing container on a towel to remove moisture from bottom of pan. Wait 1 minute and stir in essential oils or flavorings.

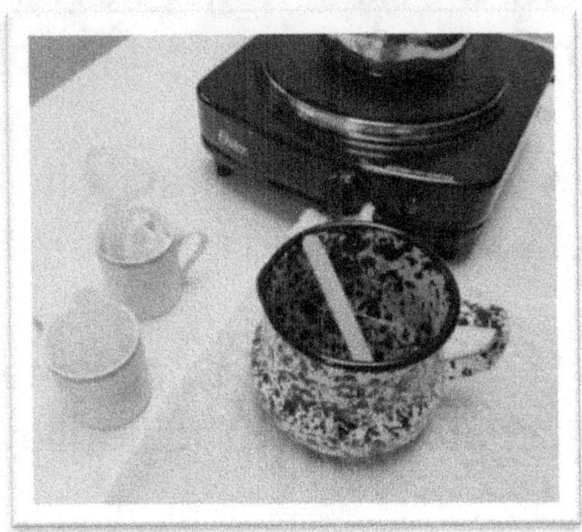

4. Pour into containers or tubes.

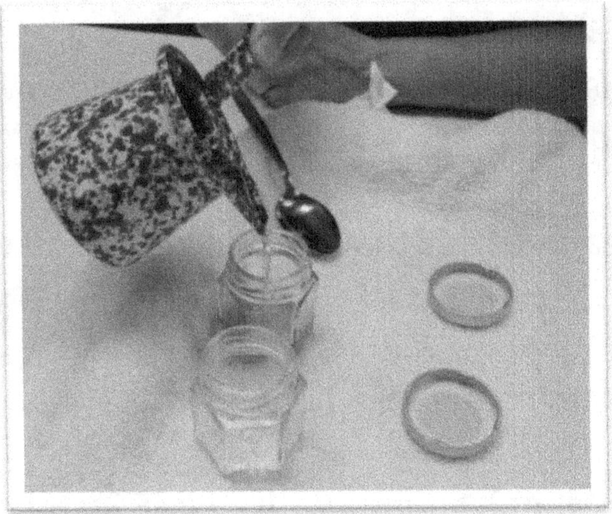
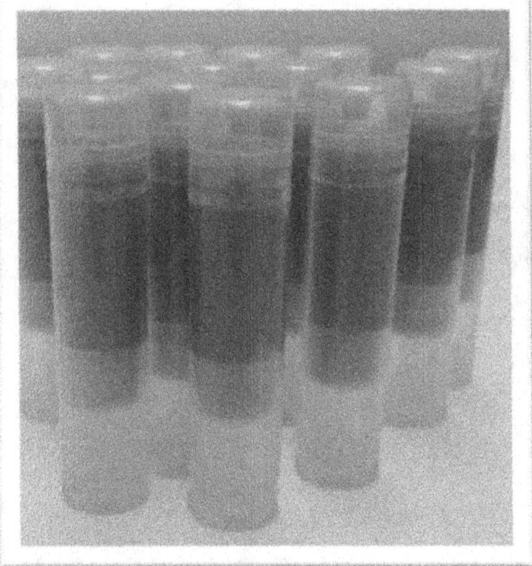

5. Let cool completely before capping.
6. Use rubbing alcohol to clean the outside of your product before labeling with ingredients.

Adding Honey to Salve and Lip Balm Recipes

Honey is an emollient, it is soothing and a humectant, (retains moisture) to help hydrate the skin. Honey has its' own healing properties. So, of course you want to add it to your salve or lip balm.

You cannot believe how much more hydrating lip balm is to your lips with the honey, or applied to chapped and chafed skin.

 Although you may find many recipes adding honey to salve or lip balm recipes, the honey will separate out without follow additional instructions.

The recipe will have to be emulsified by constantly stirring it until the salve has thickened and cooled.

Honey is not fat soluble. Honey is water soluble and will only dissolve in water or other water like liquid.

Honey will work in lotion and cream recipes that contain water and use an emulsifier.

Remember the bees use beeswax to contain the honey.

For extra healing properties use Manuka honey with a UMF factor of 10 or more.

Honey Salve Recipe

Honey Propolis Salve

1-2 tablespoons of beeswax;
1 tablespoon will make a more runny salve and 2 tablespoons will make a firmer salve.

5 tablespoons of oil infused with propolis

1 teaspoon of honey

Optional: up to 20 drops of essential oil

1-2 tablespoons of beeswax
5 tablespoons of propolis infused oil

1 teaspoon of honey
Optional: up to 20 drops of essential oil

1. Melt the beeswax.

2. Add the oil and honey and stir until the oil and honey is liquid and mixed into the beeswax.

3. Stir in the optional essential oils.

4. Remove from heat and stir constantly until the salve is thickened and cool.

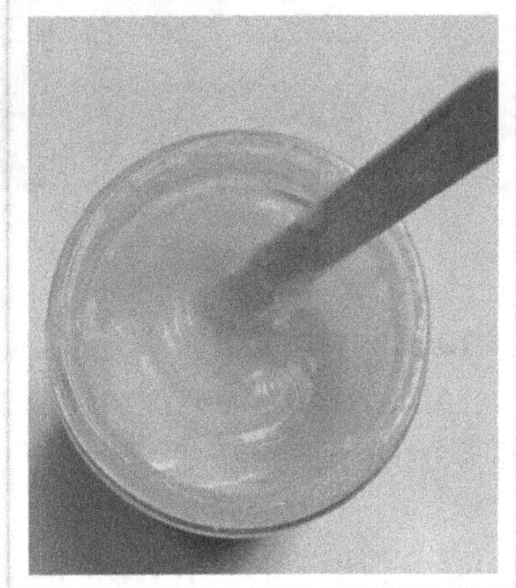

5. You may divide the salve into smaller containers. This obviously will not work in the lip balm tubes.

Castor Oil and Menthol Crystals

Castor oil is treated differently when trying to make a salve or an ointment.
It is very thick and has a long shelf life. It is often combined with beeswax to make a non petroleum jelly.

When mixing castor oil and beeswax you will need to melt them both in a separate container. You cannot add cold castor oil to the melted beeswax. You cannot melt them together.

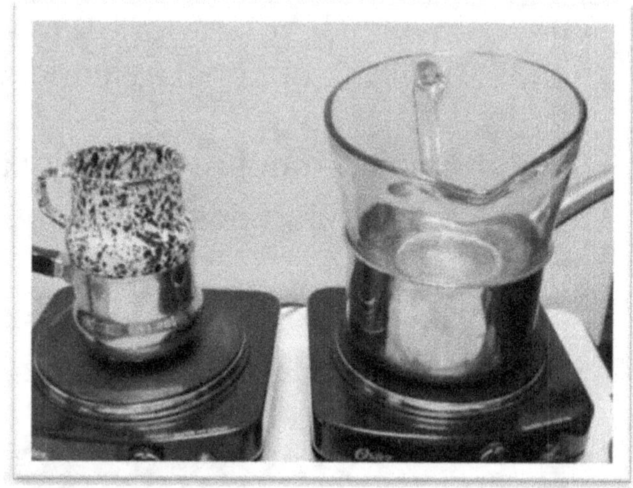

About Menthol Crystals:
Menthol crystals are made with the essential oil of corn mint. The essential oil is frozen at -22 degrees f., which turns it into crystals.

These crystals will dissolve in water or oil at 111.2 degrees f. These are very cooling and are used in everything from mouthwash, to pain relieving gel, shampoos and throat sprays. This is one time you must use a thermometer.

Castor Oil Menthol Rub

<table>
<tr><td>

Castor Oil Menthol Rub

Weigh
90 grams of Castor oil
9 grams of beeswax
1 gram of Vitamin E
3 grams of menthol crystals

Optional: for a stronger blend add 15 drops of essential oil Peppermint,
Do not use this stronger blend on children.

Instead of essential oil of peppermint use my Sinus Blend: Mix equal amounts of the essential oils of peppermint, lavender and eucalyptus.

</td><td>

1. Weigh:
90 grams of castor oil or castor oil infused with propolis
9 grams of beeswax
1 gram of vitamin E
3 grams of menthol crystal

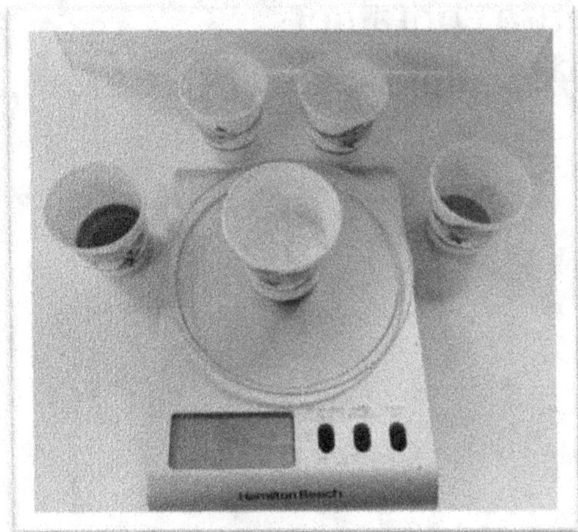

2. Heat the castor oil in the smaller container and keep warm. Usually turning off the heat and leaving it sitting over the double boiler with hot water will keep it warm.

3. Melt the beeswax in the larger container.

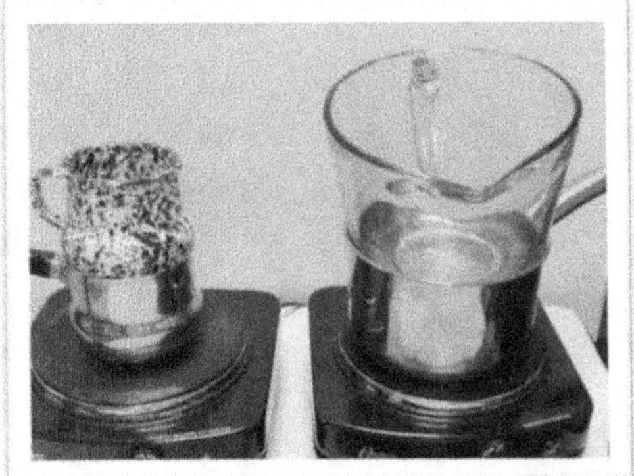

</td></tr>
</table>

4. Remove from heat.

5. Stir the warm castor oil into the beeswax.

6. Use a thermometer to make sure the mixture is at least 112 ° f. Place back on the double boiler if necessary to bring up the temperature. Remove from the heat once that temperature is reached.

7. Stir in the menthol crystals.

8. Stir in the Vitamin E.

9. Stir in the optional essential oil.

10. Pour into containers.

11. Let it completely cool before capping and labeling.

LOTIONS AND CREAMS

 For everyday use you might not like the consistency of salves. Lotions and creams have added water to them, up to 50-75% water, therefore do not contain as much as your healing ingredients like propolis.

Oils and beeswax do not promote the growth of bacteria and mold. They do however require an antioxidant to prevent the oil from going rancid. If you are making propolis oil, the propolis itself may prevent the oil from going rancid. Of course the question is "how much propolis in the oil is enough?" That would of course depend on the oil used and how much heat and oxygen was it exposed to. Without chemical analysis of the oil, just add Vitamin E to be sure. Make your products in small containers. Every time the container is opened it is being exposed to oxygen which causes oxidation.

Water promotes the growth of mold and bacteria. If you are making a lotion or a cream you are adding water and therefore need to add a preservative or keep it refrigerated. You will also still need to use vitamin E to keep the product from going rancid.

Water and oil do not mix. Beeswax is not an emulsifier. It is a thickener. If you use recipes that contain water, the water will eventually separate out. Emulsifying wax is used to blend or emulsify water and oil together. Emulsifying wax can be either plant based or petroleum based. Ask your supplier. My book "Handmade from the Hive" has recipes for lotions that have honey and propolis in it.

If you do not want to use a preservative or emulsifying wax, you might prefer to make lotion bars.

Lotion bars are solid lotion. They do not contain water. They are basically equal amounts of beeswax, oil and nut butter. A firmer bar can be made by adding a higher percentage of beeswax.

Lotion Bar Recipe #1

Weigh 8 oz. Beeswax
Weigh 8 oz. Shea Butter
Weigh 8 oz. of oil infused with propolis

1. Melt the beeswax first in top of the double boiler.

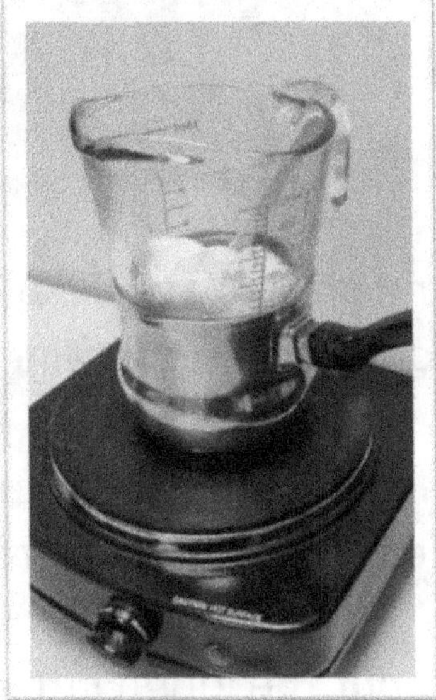

Lotion Bar Recipe # 1

8 oz. by weight Beeswax
8 oz. by weight Shea Butter or other nut butter of your choice.
8 oz. by weight oil infused with propolis
¾ teaspoon of Vitamin E
½ - 1 teaspoon of essential oil

Small Recipe:
1 tablespoon of beeswax
1 tablespoon of shea butter
1 tablespoon of oil infused with propolis
½ teaspoon of Vitamin E
10-20 drops essential oils

2. Add the oils and butter and melt together.

I have used a heat proof measuring glass on top of a small pan. Have a towel nearby to set the measuring cup on to dry the bottom of the cup. If you drip water into your lotion or your molds, it may cause the mixture to seize up.

3. Remove from the heat; wait about 1 minute before adding your vitamin E and essential oils.

4. Pour into molds and let set 10-15 minutes.

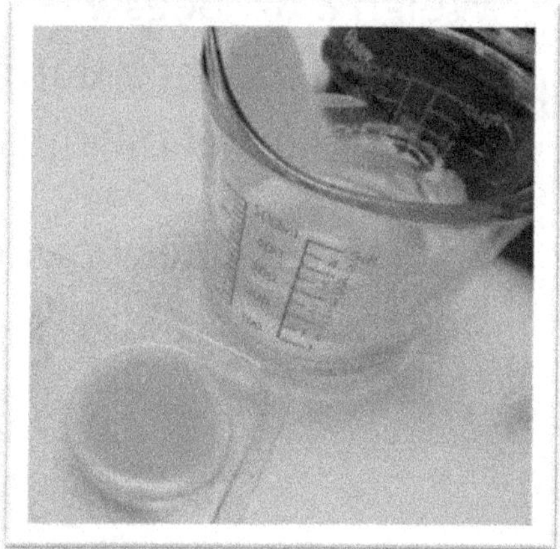

5. Pour out and place on wax paper to continue to cool. When completely cool place in container.

Optional: Place the mold in the refrigerator to set the lotion bar quicker and for easier removal from the mold.

You can also pour the lotion into a deodorant container or tube, making it a roll on lotion.

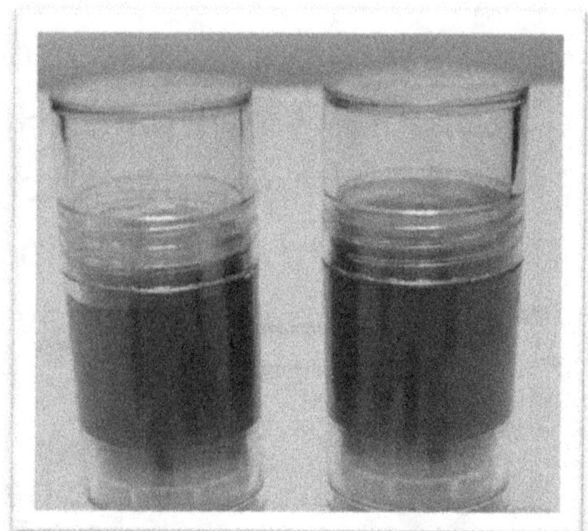

Let these cool completely before putting on the lid.

**Lotion Bar
Recipe # 2**

Measure:

2/3 cup of Beeswax

½ cup of Coconut oil infused with propolis

½ cup of Cocoa Butter

1 teaspoon of Vitamin E

45 drops of essential oil

Small Recipe:
1 tablespoon of Beeswax
1 tablespoon of Cocoa Butter
1 tablespoon of Coconut Oil
½ teaspoon of Vitamin E
10 - 20 drops of essential oils

Lotion Bar Recipe # 2

Notice: More beeswax in the recipe. Makes a firmer lotion bar.

Measure:
2/3 cup of Beeswax
½ cup of Coconut Oil infused with propolis
½ cup of Cocoa Butter

1. Melt the beeswax first in top of the double boiler.

2. Add the coconut oil and the cocoa butter and melt together.

3. Remove from the heat; place the container on a towel to remove the moisture from the bottom.

4. Wait 1 minute and then add the Vitamin E and the essential oils. If making the smaller recipe do not wait, go ahead and add the essential oils and vitamin E now.

5. Pour into the molds or tubes.

6. If using molds, wait 10-15 minutes to remove from the molds, or place in the refrigerator to set up quicker.

7. Let them set on wax or parchment paper to cool completely before placing in a container.

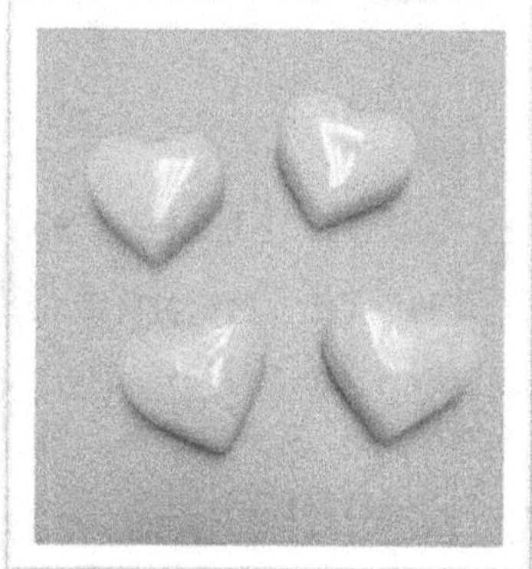

8. If using the tubes, let them cool completely before placing on the lid.

6 Guide to Using Honey and Propolis Remedies

Honey and Propolis are awesome healers. They do sometimes need a little help from their friends, herbs.

Many herbs such as garlic, ginger, cinnamon, thyme, turmeric and oregano are in your nearby grocery store.
Herbs such as peppermint, chamomile and lemon balm are easily available in the herb tea department.

Remedies: Anti-inflammatory and Joint Pain

Honey:

Honey acts as a diuretic and removes excess water from tissues and joints relieving inflammation.
Take 2-3 teaspoons of honey a day to be effective for inflammation.
This can easily be accomplished by substituting honey as your sweetener throughout the day.

For honey to be effective you may need to take it for up to 4-6 weeks to start feeling results.

Remember this is not a religion. If you are in extreme pain , if you have been doing strenuous or unfamiliar exercise or activity, you may need to see a doctor for a temporary prescription or you may need to use an over the counter pain reliever such as Ibuprofen or Tylenol.

If you are diabetic and cannot have honey, then propolis may be a better choice for you.

Adding finely chopped or powdered herbs to the honey would enhance this effect.
Turmeric, cinnamon, and chamomile are some of the suggested herbs for inflammation.
Even though Chamomile is mostly known as an herb to help one sleep and digestive complaints it is also for inflammation.
Turmeric reduces inflammation throughout the body especially the gastrointestinal tract, although it is being used for joint pain.
A few drops of the essential oil of Boswellia, known as Frankincense added to a spoon of honey will also help with inflammation.

Having Herbal Infused Honey, Herbal Honey Syrup, or Oxymels is a nice alternative to teas or pills and for those who cannot have alcohol based tinctures or extracts. See chapter 3.

 Herbal Elixirs are a combination of alcohol based tinctures or extracts that are combined with honey.

Turmeric Herbal Honey, Herbal Honey Syrup, Oxymel, or Elixir Dosage:

1 teaspoon of infused honey or honey syrup throughout the day for an adult. If you are taking the tincture add ¼ teaspoon of tincture to a spoon of honey. Turmeric works better if a pinch of black pepper is added.

Child' Dosage: An adult dosage is based on a 150 lb adult. Divide the 150 by the child's weight.
Example: A 50 lb child would be 1/3 of 150 making the dose 1/3 of a teaspoon.

Propolis:
Propolis has been called an all natural aspirin.   The bioflavonoids in propolis block or inhibit the same enzymes as aspirins that produce prostaglandins which causes the inflammation and fever.

All propolis is not alike. Propolis gathered from tropical regions does not always have the important phytochemical: caffeic acid phenethyl ester (CAPE) which is responsible for the anti-inflammatory property of propolis.

Assuming you have propolis from a non tropical source, you would need to take 3-5 grams of propolis a day, or 3-5 droppers full of a propolis tincture. This will take 4-6 weeks to feel the results. After 4-6 weeks you can reduce your dosage by half. A dropper full is 30 drops.

If you have acute conditions you would need to use 4-7 grams a day or 4-7 dropper full for 3-6 days.

HEALING REMEDIES: ANTI- SPASMODIC

Anti-spasmodic herbs work by easing tension in the muscles of the body. Different herbs are better for the muscles of the respiratory system such as coughs, muscles of the skeleton system such as muscle tension and cramps, the reproduction system such as ovarian cramps and the digestive system such as relieving gas and cramps.

These herbs can be made into a tea sweetened with honey, taken as an herbal infused honey, syrup, or oxymel.

Respiratory System: these are herbs that will help relieve spasmodic coughs.
Aniseed, California Poppy, Garlic, Thyme, Valerian, Wild Cherry

Digestive System: Herbs that will help relieve gas and cramps
1 drop of the essential oil of Basil into 1 teaspoon of honey added to 1 cup of hot water and drink.
Or
Make a tea with fresh Basil and add honey and drink.
Make a Peppermint tea and add honey.
Make a tea with Chamomile and add honey.
Crystallized Ginger or Ginger tea with honey.

Add the essential oils of Basil or Peppermint to a salve or lotion and rub on the belly.

Reproductive System and Muscles of the Skeleton: helps ease ovarian cramps and tense muscle and cramps.

Even though Black Cohosh and Wild Yam's claim to fame is as a women's herb it is also for spasms.

Others would be Black Haw, Cramp Bark, Lemon Balm, Chamomile, California Poppy, Valerian, Lavender and St. John's Wort. Some of these herbs, especially Valerian, would not be so tasty if made into a tea or added to honey.   Lemon Balm, Chamomile, Lavender and California Poppy would make tasty teas:

REMEDIES: BEE AND WASP STINGS:

While many books and references may say that honey will relieve bee and wasp stings we find propolis tincture is the most effective.

We keep it in a roll on bottle and in a spray bottle.

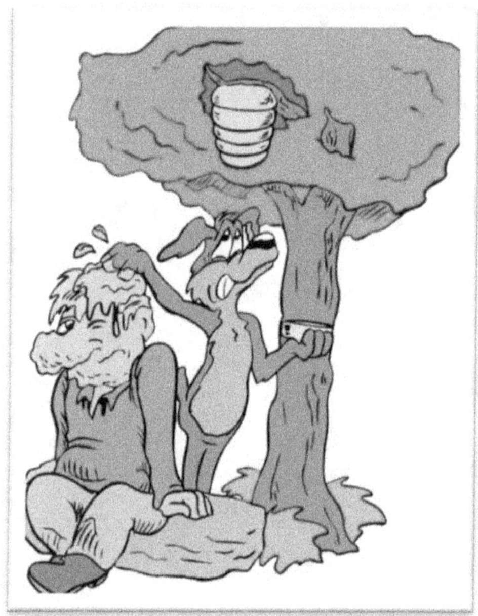

HEALING REMEDIES: BURNS

First cool off the area. You do not want anything to hold in the heat and continue the burn.

Dip in cool water, optional: add apple cider vinegar to the water, or
Apply a diluted apple cider vinegar compress, or

Use the Aloe, Lavender Spray:
2 oz. amber or blue bottle with spray lid
1 fl oz of Aloe Vera Juice
30 drops of essential oil of Lavender
Mix together, cap and store in the refrigerator.
Shake well and spray directly on burns to cool off the burned area.

Honey:
Apply honey directly on the burned area after the area has been cooled. Reapply after 30 minutes if necessary.

Larger areas will require bandaging the area and taping off the area to prevent the honey from seeping out.
Apply honey to a pad of gauze thickly,
Place on burn,
Add more gauze pads to take up the leaking honey,
Tape down on all sides to prevent the honey from leaking out.

Honey immediately seals off the burned tissue from air to reduce the pain. Honey will moisturize the area, will act as antiseptic preventing infections and start the healing process.
Optional: add essential oil of Lavender to the honey.

Caution about using essential oils:
Regardless of how effective they are they can burn.

Propolis:

I would use honey at first which will allow the burn "to breathe".
Propolis oil or a salve would tend to hold the heat in.
 Apply propolis oil or salve once the burn has started to heal.
Optional: you might add a little propolis tincture to the honey. Propolis tincture would mix with the honey, although it could burn. The propolis oil will not mix with the honey.

Caution: 3rd degree burns require medical attention. The Medihoney products for burns may be needed.

Symptoms of burns:

First degree: reddening of the skin
Second degree: Reddening of the skin and blisters
Third degree: Blisters with deeper tissue damage.

Burns on the roof of mouth from hot drink or food:
Combine Slippery Elm Powder or Marshmallow Root Powder and honey into a ball and suck on for relief.

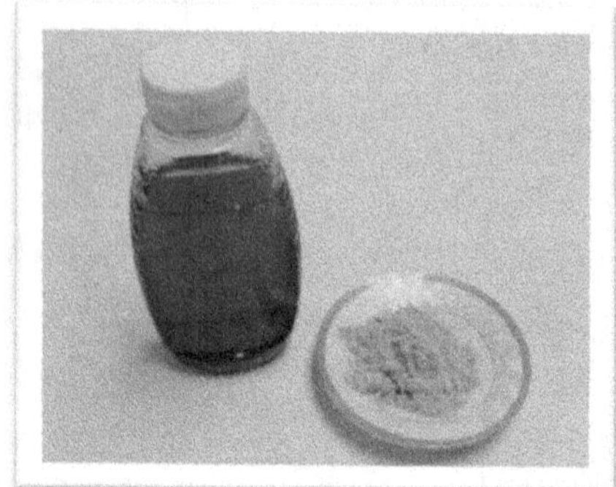
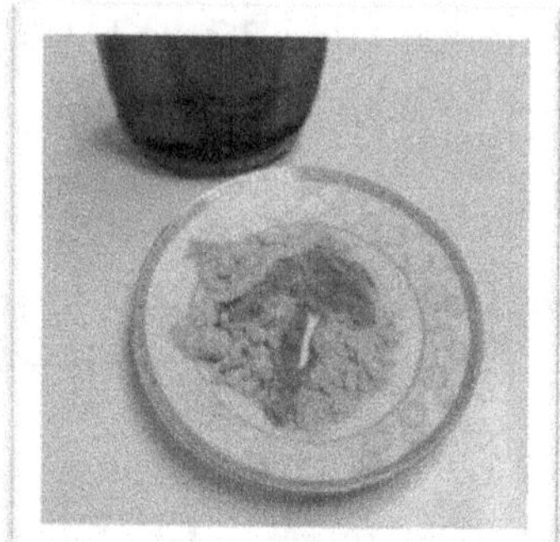
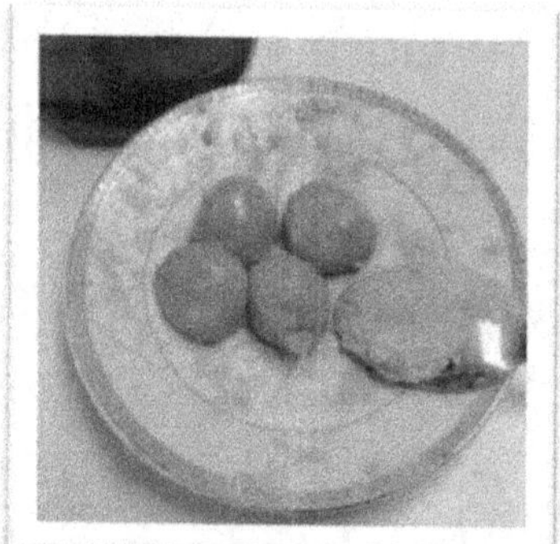

HEALING REMEDIES: COUGHS AND SORE THROAT

Coughs can be divided into 2 categories.
Coughs with mucus: the body is trying to get rid of the mucus.
Coughs without mucus: dry and irritating or spasmodic.

Honey will help both conditions.   Many herbs will work as both an antispasmodic and as an expectorant. Natural remedies are amazing as they have the ability to adapt to be whichever the body needs.
There are other things you can do to help relieve your symptoms.

Taking both propolis and honey may help prevent infection.

Coughs with mucus:
The body is trying to get rid of the mucus.
Your mission is to thin the mucus to make it easier to cough up.
You need expectorants. These do not make you cough. They thin the mucus to make it easier to cough up.

You do not need a cough suppressant or anti-spasmodic. You are trying to get the mucus out of your system.

Gargle:
Add propolis tincture to a little warm water and gargle. If you do not have a propolis tincture a salt water rinse will help. (8 oz. of water to a ¼ -1/2 teaspoon of salt).
You can also use the above as a throat spray.
Spray the throat with a propolis spray.

Plenty of hot liquids to thin the mucus.

Hot chicken soup
Any spicy food will help thin mucus.
Coffee with honey.
Peppermint or Ginger tea with honey.
Crystallized honey or ginger infused honey.
Essential oil of peppermint added to infused propolis oil rubbed on the throat and the chest.
If you do not have infused propolis, add the essential oil of peppermint to any lotion or oil that you have on hand.

Your own mix of propolis infused castor oil with menthol crystals.
If you have none of these go for the Vicks!

Mix 3 drops of essential oil of peppermint with 2 tablespoons of honey. Place a pea size of this on the back of the tongue. The molecules of the essential oil of peppermint can go behind the pharynx into the nasal cavities as a decongestant.

Mix essential oil of peppermint or my sinus blend with honey to use as a cough syrup.
Sinus Blend: equal amounts of the essential oils of peppermint, eucalyptus and lavender.

Take Elderberry Syrup throughout the day. See chapter 3.
Take the Garlic Cider Vinegar or Ginger Oxymel.
Coughs:
Add ¼ teaspoon of lemon juice or lime juice or apple cider vinegar to 1 teaspoon of honey or herbal honey such as thyme or elderberries to 1/8 oz cup of water or take straight
Take 4 times a day or as needed

Coughs without Mucus
Use an anti-spasmodic to suppress a cough or demulcent to soothe a
dry throat

Honey by itself has been proven to be more effective than cough syrups
containing dextromethorphan or diphenhydramine.
Honey will both coat the throat and act as an anti-spasmodic.

Take Elderberry Syrup, Onion Syrup or Garlic Syrup, chapter 3
Take 1 teaspoon throughout the day.

Drink herbal teas with honey.
1 teaspoon of the dried herb
1 cup of water
Honey to taste
Bring 1 cup of water almost to a boil.
Pour over the dried herbs, cover and steep 5-6 minutes.
Sweetened with honey to taste.

Suggested antispasmodic herbs:
Anise Seed
California Poppy
Thyme is an herb that is both an expectorant and antispasmodic.
Valerian (caution: unpleasant smell and taste)
Wild Cherry Bark

Slippery Elm and Licorice Root are demulcents that will help coat the
throat. Chapter 3
Use the Slippery Elm Throat Soothers
Make an herbal infused honey with the above herbs.

Take 1 teaspoon of an herbal honey or other honey remedy throughout the day for an adult.

Optional: Add a teaspoon of herb infused honey to a little yogurt or other fermented food. Research is proving that our immune system begins in the gut.

Child' Dosage: An adult dosage is based on a 150 lb adult. Divide the 150 by the child's weight.

Example: A 50 lb child would be 1/3 of 150 making the dose 1/3 of a teaspoon.

Honey Herbal Syrups see chapter 3: How to Make Honey Herbal Syrup.

There are 2 type of honey herbal syrup. One recipe can be made in an hour's time. It must be refrigerated and used in a couple of weeks or frozen.

The other type of honey herbal syrup is made by combining an herb infused honey with a concentrated herb infusion and an herb tincture or extract.

Bronchitis and whooping cough

1 tablespoon of honey with 1 teaspoon of finely chopped thyme

Thyme infused honey or honey herbal syrup.

Take 1 teaspoon of an herbal honey or other honey remedy throughout the day for an adult.

Child' Dosage: An adult dosage is based on a 150 lb adult. Divide the 150 by the child's weight.

Example: A 50 lb child would be 1/3 of 150 making the dose 1/3 of a teaspoon.

PPC: Persistent Post-Infectious Cough
Drink coffee with honey. A study in Iran showed coffee with honey to be as effective as prednisolone and guaifenesin.
Mix an equal amount of prepared coffee with honey.

Sore Throat:
2 teaspoons of raw honey
1 teaspoon of apple cider vinegar
Dilute with water and use as a gargle and sip throughout the day.

Add lemon juice to honey and a drop of the essential oil of eucalyptus, peppermint or my sinus blend: equal amounts of the essential oils of eucalyptus, peppermint and lavender.
Do not give this to children or pregnant women.

Spray the throat with propolis spray.

Infected Throat like Strep Throat:
If you do not have a propolis extract try garlic.

Garlic is considered nature's antibiotic. Of course most know that a cold or flu is not a bacterium so it will not respond to antibiotics. Garlic like most herbs are not an antibiotic, they are antimicrobial which means virus, fungus or bacteria.
If you are not responding to the garlic and honey treatment seek a medical professional. This is not a religion. It is the first line of defense.

Is it Strep Throat?

Strep throat is a bacterial infection, while colds and flu are viral infections, and only a test by the doctor can confirm if the infection is strep throat.

Symptoms

Sudden throat pain without coughing, sneezing, and other symptoms of a cold.

Difficulty or pain with swallowing.

Fever of 101°F. or more. A lower fever may indicate a viral infection instead of strep.

Red and swollen tonsils.

White or yellow spots or a coating on the throat and tonsils.

Bright red spots on the throat.

Dark red spots back on the roof of the mouth.

Swollen, tender lymph glands in the neck.

Fever.

Headache.

Rash.

Stomach ache and sometimes vomiting in young children.

Fatigue.

If a rough rash develops and spreads over the neck and chest and then to rest of the body this could indicate scarlet fever.

If you develop these symptoms after 1-2 weeks after the strep infection, you may have rheumatic fever **see a doctor.**

Weakness

Shortness of breath

Joint pain

Raised red rash or lumps under the skin

Uncontrolled, jerking movements of the arms or legs

When using garlic as an antibiotic or antimicrobial mince the garlic and let it set 10-15 minutes. The garlic cells must be ruptured to release two separate chemicals of the garlic, alliin and alliinase which then form a new compound called allicin.

Remember this is not a religion. See a doctor if you are not healing.

Eating too much garlic at once may cause tummy problems, so start slowly and build up.

Garlic and honey is also good for high blood pressure if taken twice everyday

REMEDIES: FOR DIGESTIVE PROBLEMS

When you are dealing with digestive issues you have to consider if it is a physical problem like a blockage or constipation, or a nervous tension problem.

Is the problem nausea, or is it caused by constipation, sinus drainage, viral infection, motion or nervous tension?   Most digestive problems will benefit from the carminative herbs such as Chamomile, Lemon Balm and California Poppy.

Irritable bowel syndrome: minimum of 3-4 teaspoons of honey a day to relieve bloating, abdominal pain, diarrhea. Adding the herbs chamomile would be more effective.

Colitis:
Dissolve 3 tablespoons of honey into a glass of lukewarm water. Drink in the evening.

Diarrhea:
Honey will not cure diarrhea overnight but will shorten the duration of the problem, rehydrate and is effective against the bacteria causing the diarrhea.

Dissolve 4 tablespoons of honey into 2 cups of warm water.
Drink throughout the day.

Add honey to yogurt. Yogurt adds friendly bacteria to the gut.
Honey is a prebiotic that feeds and supports the growth of the lactic acid bacteria.

Honey is a dual purpose remedy. It decreases the bad pathogens while increasing the beneficial bacteria in the gut.

Peptic Ulcers:
Peptic ulcers are caused by the bacteria, Helicobacter pylori. Honey is particularly effective against these bacteria.   Manuka Honey would be the most effective honey to take. Take 2-3 teaspoons of honey up to 3 times a day for several weeks for relief.

Nausea and upset stomach
Few drops of the essential oil of Peppermint added to honey. Take as needed.
Peppermint tea, gum or candy.

Nausea due to motion or sinus drainage
Crystallized ginger
Ginger Infused Honey or ginger added to honey
Ginger Oxymel
Ginger Syrup, Chapter 3 How to Make Honey Herbal Syrup.
1 teaspoon throughout the day for an adult.
Child' Dosage: An adult dosage is based on a 150 lb adult. Divide the 150 by the child's weight.
Example: A 50 lb child would be 1/3 of 150 making the dose 1/3 of a teaspoon.

Caution: Ginger may be too spicy for some or cause heartburn. Peppermint would then be your herb of choice.

REMEDIES: EAR ACHE AND SWIMMER'S EAR

Warm a bottle of propolis oil in a cup of warm water. Add a few drops of propolis to the ear. Use a cotton ball to prevent the propolis oil from leaking out.

Swimmer's Ear: Place several drops of propolis tincture into the ear. Turn the ear so that the tincture runs out.

If you have propolis tincture in a roll on bottle, roll the tincture around the outside of the ear and the glands in the throat.

Hard of Hearing or Titinitus: May help some people.
Drop propolis oil into the ear canal and plug the ears with cotton.
Repeat for 2-3 days. Do this 9 times throughout the month.
If you do not see improvement in a month's time this may not work for you.

REMEDIES: EYE INFECTIONS AND STIES

The eyes must be treated with clean hands.

A saline eye wash can be used to thoroughly clean the eyes.
Saline Eye Wash:
Dissolve ½ teaspoon of salt into 1 cup of boiling distilled water.
Pour into clean container and let cool before using.
Replace each day.

Apply honey directly to the eyelids for bumps and sores on the eye lids such as sties. If you get the honey on the inside of the eye, it will sting but will not be harmful.

Using 2-3 drops of liquid honey in the eyes is used in countries such as Nigeria to prevent cataracts.

If you have been to the eye doctor and were told that you have Blepharitis and were prescribed an eye salve, honey may be another solution. I have used these salves which you apply at bedtime and then it is almost impossible to wash it off your eyes the next morning causing difficulty seeing.

Blepharitis is a common eye condition that causes eye lid inflammation. There are two types of Blepharitis, anterior Blepharitis which is caused by bacteria and posterior Blepharitis which affects the inner eyelid and is caused by oil glands in this part of the eyelid. Skin disorders such as acne, rosacea and scalp dandruff can also cause posterior blepharitis.

Anterior Blepharitis is caused by the bacteria Staphylococcus and scalp dandruff. Since honey is effective against Staphylococcus you might try honey instead of the salve. I apply the honey to my eyelids every morning when I wash my face. I let it sit for about 30 minutes and then wash my eyelids. You could also do this routine at night. Optional: Mix equal amounts of distilled water with honey and apply to the eyelids.

If the Blepharitis is caused by dandruff, use a dandruff shampoo on your hair or do a honey rinse when you wash your hair. Add enough water to honey to apply to your hair, leave on 15-30 minutes and then rinse.

Blepharitis is a chronic condition and must be treated for a lifetime.

Conjunctivitis
Conjunctivitis can be a bacterial or viral infection or allergic conjunctivitis.
Apply honey directly to the eyelids. Leave on for 30 minutes and rinse.
Optional: Mix equal amounts of distilled water and honey and apply to the eyelids. Do this several times during the day.

Honey Eye Drops:

Boil 1 cup of distilled water with a pinch of salt. Let cool, but still warm enough to dissolve a ¼ teaspoon of raw or Manuka honey. Let cool to room temperature.
Either use a cotton ball to rub around the eyes or a clean eye dropper 1-2 drops 3 times a day.

Prepare fresh each day.

REMEDIES: DENTAL AND GUM

Propolis extract sprayed in the mouth or added to a little water as a mouth rinse relieves the inflammation and heals mouth sores and gum problems. Take a dropper full (30 drops) 4 times a day.

Mix baking soda or bentonite clay with propolis oil or tincture to use as toothpaste.

I have seen many recipes using coconut oil. I am a big fan of coconut oil. But not in my sink.

Keep in mind, coconut oil becomes a solid when the temperature is below 76° f., this could become a problem stopping up your plumbing.

We put coconut oil in our coffee. We are careful to always pour leftover coffee in the yard and not down the drain.

 Harmful substances in commercial toothpaste:

Triclosan: a pesticide and hormone disruptor
Sodium lauryl sulfate: may cause canker sores in some people
Fluoride: can be toxic and does not work in toothpaste
Titanium dioxide: added to toothpaste to make it white. Even though most data shows it is safe, studies have not been done to show how it is absorbed by oral tissues.
Artificial coloring: linked to ADHD and hyperactivity
Glycerin: This is a great ingredient in skin care but not in the mouth. Glycerin is a soap that strips your body's natural oral mucosa and leaves a film. This film may could alter the microbiome in the mouth and impact the natural re-mineralization process.

Highly abrasive ingredients: damages the tooth enamel, making teeth more sensitive and more prone to gum recession and cavities.

Better abrasives:
Baking soda is alkaline and would neutralize acids that breakdown enamel.
Bentonite clay is a natural polisher, rich in minerals that is not too abrasive and is also alkaline.

REMEDIES: HAY FEVER

Is it a drip, drip, drip, or, are you drowning in your mucus?

Preventing hay fever should be your first step. When you know that you have been exposed to pollen, dust or other irritants, clean your nose with a saline solution with a neti pot, a syringe or a nasal spray bottle.

A homemade version of the saline solution:
3 heaping teaspoons of salt: with no iodine or preservative
1 teaspoon of baking soda: to buffer the salt
Container to store the salt solution
1 cup of boiled distilled water

Mix the salt and baking soda together.
Store in a clean container and label.
Add 1 teaspoon of this mixture to the cup of hot water. Cool to lukewarm.
Optional: Add 1 dropper full of propolis tincture
Irrigate the nose several times a day.
If you cannot do this, at least wet a cloth and use the corner to clean out your nose.

Take at least one teaspoon of honey from your region a day. For those who really suffer from hay fever, pollen capsules might work better, at least 3-5 capsules a day.

Another alternative is to mix pollen with the honey. Much of the bee pollen cannot be digested by the human body. Bee pollen has a hard outer coat that we cannot digest. Grinding up the pollen breaks down this coat and soaking it in honey furthers softens the pollen making it more available to us.

Apply the honey propolis salve to relieve your sore chapped nose from constantly wiping your nose.

Taking honey and pollen works great for many people most of the time. There are those times it does not seem to be working. Maybe it is not pollen at all but some other irritants. Then you might need some herbal help.

I do eat honey everyday and also take 2 stinging nettle leaf capsules a day to prevent hay fever. Stinging nettle leaf is for general all round allergies. Use the stinging nettle leaf not the root. The roots are used for prostrate problems.

 I also make a ragweed tincture.   A ragweed tincture is especially effective for the runny nose type hay fever caused by ragweed, and juniper berries would be more effective for allergies caused by cedar pollen. Instead of making a tincture you could also make an infused honey or oxymel.

Take 1 teaspoon of an herbal honey or other honey remedy throughout the day for an adult.
Child' Dosage: An adult dosage is based on a 150 lb adult. Divide the 150 by the child's weight.
Example: A 50 lb child would be 1/3 of 150 making the dose 1/3 of a teaspoon.
If taking the tincture or extract take ¼ teaspoon,

Golden Rod is another one of the herbs for treating the symptoms of hay fever. Because it grows and blooms the same time as Ragweed it often gets the blame. Golden Rod's pollen is too large to create problems. Ragweed's pollen is very small and easily blown about by the wind and easily inhaled.

Golden Rod will act as both an antihistamine and a decongestant. It is especially good for nasal congestion due to allergies, cold or the flu. Make this into a tea sweetened with honey, Herbal Infused Honey, or Honey Herbal Syrup, chapter 3.

Herbs that reduce excessive mucus:
Elderflowers, not the berries combined with peppermint
Yarrow
Echinacea

REMEDIES: HEART TONIC

Honey contains tiny amounts of acetylcholine which helps transmit nerve impulses throughout the body. Take 2-3 teaspoons of honey 30 minutes before bedtime for 2-3 weeks. Your heart rate should drop and become more stable.

Combine honey with ground cinnamon to spread on toast, add to oatmeal or yogurt. Add hawthorn berries to this mix for its heart healthy benefits.

Cinnamon is best known as a digestive aid. Cassia cinnamon is used to help lower blood sugar levels in diabetics.   Take approximately 1 teaspoon a day in divided doses to be effective.

 Cinnamon has a small amount of coumarin acting as a blood thinner increasing circulation. Large amounts of cinnamon should be avoided a week before surgery. Large amounts of cinnamon may be harmful for those who suffer from liver problems.

Herbs that are taken daily as a tonic or to treat a chronic condition do not have to be treated as a medicine. They are very well suited to being added to treats or a nutritional snack. One of my favorite treats is Honey Protein Hawthorn Balls that I add powdered Hawthorn berries.

 Hawthorn berries are one of the most recognized herbs for the heart. It helps keep the heart healthy by strengthening the force at which the heart muscle beats, helps maintain normal heart rhythm and improves blood flow. It lowers blood pressure and cholesterol. As an antioxidant it is used to fight free radicals. All of this being said, if you have a serious heart condition do not substitute Hawthorn berries for your heart medication without medical advice.

Since it is nutrition for the heart it must be taken daily in adequate amounts. Recommended amount is ¼ teaspoon 3 times a day.

Add ¼ teaspoon of powdered hawthorn berries and honey to taste to your morning oatmeal or to unsweetened yogurt.

Another combination that is good for the heart would be making an herbal honey, herbal honey syrup, or oxymel from equal amounts of Lemon Balm, Hawthorn berries, and Turmeric.   Adding a pinch of black pepper will help the body better absorb Turmeric.
Hawthorn berries and Turmeric are good for the heart and Lemon Balm helps reduce blood pressure that is due to tension.

These Honey Protein Energy Balls can be eaten as a treat or as a quick breakfast food.

Honey Protein Energy Balls

1 ¼ cups of old fashion oats

3 Tablespoons of shredded coconut

½ cup of chopped almonds, walnuts or other nuts

1 heaping tablespoon of powdered hawthorn berries

1 scoop of whey protein powder or your choice of other protein powder

1 teaspoon of powdered cinnamon and other spices you desire. Optional: your favorite pumpkin pie spices.

½ cup of honey

½ cup of almond butter or peanut butter.

½ cup of chopped dried apricots

In one bowl combine the oats, coconut, chopped nuts, powdered Hawthorn berries and protein powder and optional spices. Stir well. In another bowl combine the honey and nut butter together. Combine this with the dry ingredients. Add the chopped apricots. You may need to use your hands to evenly distribute all ingredients. Chill in the refrigerator for about 20 – 30 minutes. Scoop out and then roll into balls. Keep refrigerated, will last about a week.

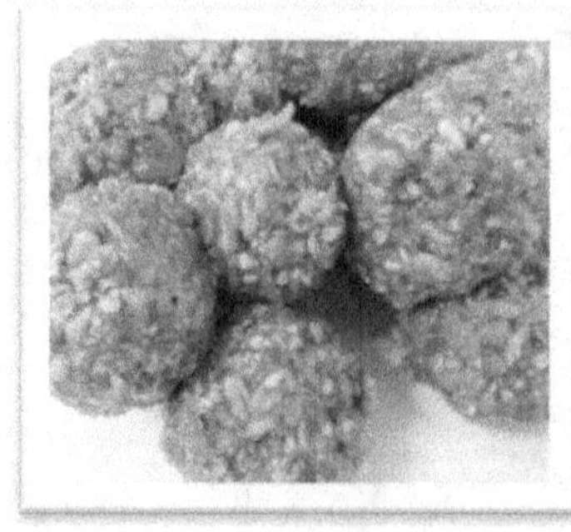

REMEDIES: HERPES, COLD SORES & GENITAL HERPES

Cold Sores: Apply honey directly to the cold sore, or a propolis tincture, oil, or salve.

Genital Herpes:

Studies show a combination of beeswax, olive oil infused with propolis and honey effective in relieving genital herpes. Making the Honey Propolis Salve using Manuka Honey would be especially effective. See chapter 5.

This mixture was applied 4 times a day. Results were seen in as little as 3 days and took up to 10 days for others.

Like all medications, there was not 100% cure. Relief was seen in about 75% of the study participants.

REMEDIES: IMPETIGO

Impetigo appears as red sores on the face of infants and children that burst and develop honey colored crusts. The sores are highly contagious and may clear up on their own in 2-3 weeks. As long as there are sores it is infectious. Antibiotics will shorten the duration of the sores and will help prevent it infecting other children.

Honey for Impetigo: Try a diluted honey wash twice a day. Add enough water to honey to make a wash.

Remedies: Itchy Skin

Many times itchy skin is due to dryness.
Apply the Honey Propolis Salve or Propolis Oil or one of the Lotion Bars.

REMEDIES: INSOMNIA AND NERVOUS TENSION

Honey contains acetylcholine which acts as a chemical transmitter of nerve impulses. Not only good for the heart but all nerve conditions.

Nutmeg, Honey and Milk:
8 oz. of milk or milk alternative
1 tablespoon of honey
¼ teaspoon of nutmeg (freshly grated is the best)
Warm milk and nutmeg in a small saucepan. Remove from heat, add honey and stir.
Drink an hour before bedtime.

Honey supplies fuel to the liver throughout the night that so you are not woke up by the liver.
Honey activates the production of melatonin and serotonin.
Honey releases tryptophan in the brain.

Nutmeg is a natural muscle relaxant.
Nutmeg inhibits the release of stress hormones.
Nutmeg contains magnesium, a necessary mineral for sleep.
Nutmeg helps calm a racing mind.
Caution: Take only ¼ teaspoon. Large amounts of nutmeg can cause hallucinations, vomiting, and heart palpitations and possible death.

If it is summertime and you do not want anything hot, try the honey and nutmeg over plain yogurt.

Mix ¼ teaspoon of ground nutmeg with 1- 2 tablespoons of honey.

Honey and Apple Cider Vinegar
Mix 1 teaspoon of apple cider vinegar with 1/3 cup of honey.
Take 2 teaspoons at bedtime; if still awake take another teaspoon in an hour. Keep by the bed stand. If you awake during the night take another 2 teaspoons.
Note: you do not need to take the teaspoons of honey all at one time. You could take 1 teaspoon and take another teaspoon later.

Honey with herbs:
The same herbs that are used for insomnia are also used for nervous tension.
California Poppy, Chamomile, Lavender, Lemon Balm, Passionflower optional: add 1/2 part of St. John's Wort to these.
Use these herbs (any one herb or combination) to make and take Herbal Infused Honey or Syrup, see chapter 3 or tea with honey.

All of these herbs are safe for children and the elderly in reduced doses. Do not use if pregnant without your doctor's approval. Use them singly or any combination.

Nervous Tension: 1 teaspoon of infused honey or honey syrup throughout the day for an adult. If you are taking the tincture only use ¼ teaspoon combined with a spoon of honey. (Combining a tincture with honey is called an Elixir)

Insomnia: infused honey or honey syrup, take 1 teaspoon 2 hours before bed, then take another 1 teaspoon 1 hour before bed. Take 1 teaspoon if you awake during the night.

Child' Dosage: An adult dosage is based on a 150 lb adult. Divide the 150 by the child's weight. Example: A 50 lb child would be 1/3 of 150 making the dose 1/3 of a teaspoon.

REMEDIES: ABRASIONS AND IRRITATIONS INTIMATE AREAS

Honey or Lemon Balm Infused Honey, chapter 3, can be applied directly on all mucus membrane including all intimate areas.

Propolis oil can be applied to this area.

Propolis ointment with honey.

REMEDIES AND RECIPES: POISON IVY:

The oils of poison ivy must be immediately washed off. Throw clothes in the washing machine and wash immediately.
Apply honey to the rash.

Apply propolis tincture or propolis oil.

REMEDIES: PSORIASIS, ECZEMA, DERMATITIS OF ALL KINDS, SKIN RASHES, DIAPER RASH.

Propolis Ointment or oil applied several times a day.

Remedies and Recipes for Seborrheic dermatitis
Seborrheic dermatitis is a large clump of cells that build up on the surface of the scalp. Your scalp produces natural oils called sebum. Malassezia globosa is a naturally occurring microbe that breaks down this oil into an irritant called oleic acid. The oleic acid is irritating to the cells causing an increase in cell turnover which causes the large clumps of cells to build up on the surface of the scalp.

Wash scalp twice a day with honey mixed with enough water to apply to scalp.

REMEDIES: URINARY TRACT

Golden Rod Herbal Infused Honey, Oxymel, or Herbal Honey Syrup.

How to make, see Chapter 3.

Other herbs would be juniper berries.

1 teaspoon of infused honey or honey syrup throughout the day for an adult. If you are taking the tincture only use ¼ teaspoon.

Child' Dosage: An adult dosage is based on a 150 lb adult. Divide the 150 by the child's weight.

Example: A 50 lb child would be 1/3 of 150 making the dose 1/3 of a teaspoon.

REMEDIES: THE SHINGLES

Shingles creates terrible pain and burning. When my sister had shingles the doctors offered her nothing that gave her any relief.

I had just recently bought a bottle of Manuka Honey "just in case I needed it" and started applying it to her face. She had relief in less than 5 minutes.

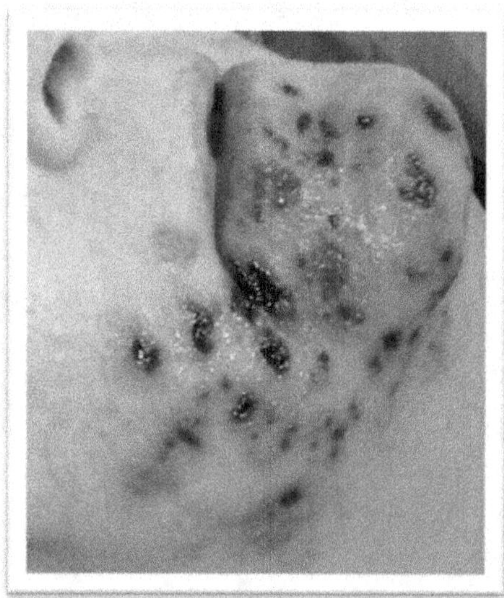

When she started to heal, she switched to propolis oil.

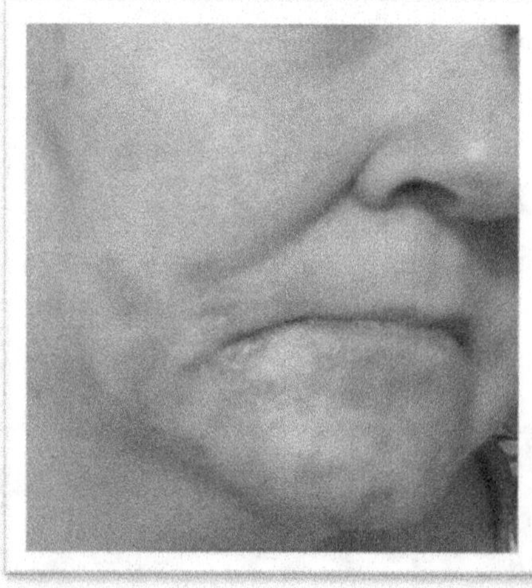

Remedies: Stuffy Nose

Even though you feel so bad you need to lie down, this may make your problem worse. All the congestion will back up in your head area. Your nose, your teeth and your jaws will ache from the pressure. Prop up your pillows to elevate your head, or sleep in your recliner.

Drink plenty of hot liquids.

A hot cup of peppermint tea with honey can start loosening things up.

Squirt warm salt water (8 oz of water with ¼ - ½ teaspoon salt) with a few drops propolis tincture inside your nose. This can be done with a neti pot, a syringe or a squirt bottle.

Squirt propolis tincture diluted with distilled water inside the nose.

When the nose is so stopped up and breathing essential oils or steam inhalation cannot penetrate try honey and the essential oil of peppermint.

 3 drops of the essential oil of peppermint
 2 tablespoons of honey.
Mix well. Place a small amount of the mixture on the back of the tongue. The molecules of the essential oil of Peppermint can go behind the pharynx into the nasal cavities as a decongestant.

Chew honeycomb or the cappings from the honeycomb. Chew a piece about the size of a stick of chewing gum. Spit out after 15 minutes.

Add the essential oil of peppermint to honeycomb as a natural chewing gum.

Try the Garlic Cider Vinegar or Ginger Oxymel.

If you grow tired of peppermint and ginger tea, or the essential oil of peppermint is just getting to be too harsh, Golden Rod is your choice. Take 1 teaspoon of Golden Rod infused honey, honey syrup or oxymel throughout the day.

Remedies Upper Respiratory:
Runny nose, sinus infection or congestion, excess mucus

Finely chop one of the herbs listed below and mix with a spoon of honey or take an Herbal Infused Honey or Honey Herbal Syrup made with these suggested herbs. See chapter 3
1 teaspoon throughout the day for an adult.
Child' Dosage: An adult dosage is based on a 150 lb adult. Divide the 150 by the child's weight.
Example: A 50 lb child would be 1/3 of 150 making the dose 1/3 of a teaspoon.

David Hoffman, herbalist, considers Golden Rod the first herb of choice for all upper respiratory conditions. Golden Rod is especially effective for sinus congestion. Golden Rod grows wild over most of the United States. There are several species of Golden Rod. If you are lucky you have the species that has an anise flavor. Here in East Texas the species we have is not the anise, but is very bitter. Early settlers and Native Americans drank the anise flavored Golden Rod as a tea and used it for its medical benefits.
Gather Golden Rod in the early fall just before the flowers open.

Hyssop is another herb for upper respiratory. I grow the anise flavored hyssop. It is the only herb I have tried that you can munch on that taste good. I often will pluck a few leaves to munch on to freshen my breath.

Dr. Christopher considers mullein the number one choice for upper respiratory conditions. Mullein is another one those plants that grow wild over much of the United States.

Used as an expectorant (thins mucus), demulcent, anti-inflammatory, anti-spasmodic, and an astringent.

Mullein leaves may be used in cough medication to control coughs and helps to loosen mucus to move it out of the body.

Mullein leaf is combined with Lobelia and Echinacea for glandular imbalances.

The herbalist, 7Song is in favor of Ragweed as a natural antihistamine.

Elderberries are not only good for runny nose and upper respiratory conditions but also can be taken at the first sign of cold or flu to prevent it. If, despite your best efforts you still get sick it has been proven to reduce the symptoms and duration or colds and the flu. Elderberries also grow wild over most of the United States. Their big cluster of white flowers can be seen from the highway in ditches and other wet areas. Take note of where they are spotted because once their flowers drop they seem to disappear. Their berries are ready to harvest in late summer or early fall.

 The Sambucol Elderberry Syrup Study Showed:
Studies showed it decreased the flu symptoms by 3-4 days
Dosage: 2-4 teaspoons ever hour or up to 1 tablespoon 4 times a day
Side effects: none
So safe you can use Elderberry syrup on your pancakes.
Source: National Geographic Guide to Medicinal Herbs and The Herbal Drugstore.

Tamiflu:
Requires a prescription
Decreases the flu by 1 day
Side effects: Mild to moderate nausea and vomiting, diarrhea, stomach pain.
Sources: Tamiflu.com and TV commercials, WebMD
Elderberry syrups are available at most drug stores and health food stores. The brand Sambucal is the brand used in the studies.

HONEY FOR WOUND CARE

A wound should first be cleaned with soap and water or a saline solution. Using honey does not take the place of cleaning the wound.

Using honey as a dressing
Fill abscesses, cavities and depressions in the wound with honey.
Cover a 4" square pad with 1 ounce of honey. If the wound is larger use a larger pad.
Cover the wound with this pad.
Place a dry pad on top of this and then bandage to keep everything in place.
Change the dressing once a day until the wound stops oozing.
If the dressing becomes saturated change more often.
 Once it stops oozing it can be changed once a week until it is healed.

Honey draws fluid and dead tissue away from the wound and into the dressing. Honey should prevent the bandage from sticking. If it does stick, use a saline solution or sterile water to moisten the bandage.

Serious wounds may require Manuka honey, or specialty products made from Manuka honey such as Medi-honey's gels and impregnated bandages available on Amazon.
Healing with honey is not a religion. If you are not seeing positive results seek medical attention.

Remedies: Warts and Corns

Warts are caused by a virus. Common warts are caused by the human papilloma virus. Warts are a signal that you need to boost your immune system.

Propolis works about 75% of the time on certain kinds of warts. Apply propolis tincture 50% strength to the warts at least 2 times a day and then cover with a bandage.
Take a dropper full of propolis tincture or 1000 mgs in capsule form at least once a day.

Warts can be very stubborn. Propolis can remove the wart in as little as 2 weeks or could take as long as 3 months.

Manuka honey can also be used. Apply Manuka honey to the wart and cover with a bandage. Do this 2 times a day. Take a teaspoon of the Manuka honey 2-3 times a day.

Corns:
Apply propolis oil or tincture to the corn and cover with a bandage. Do this 2 times a day.

7 Tips

Temporary Labels:

Painter's tape make excellent temporary labels that will stay on your jar when you need it to and come off easily when it is time to wash it.
Use a felt tip marker.
Make sure the tape does not have the brand name all over it.

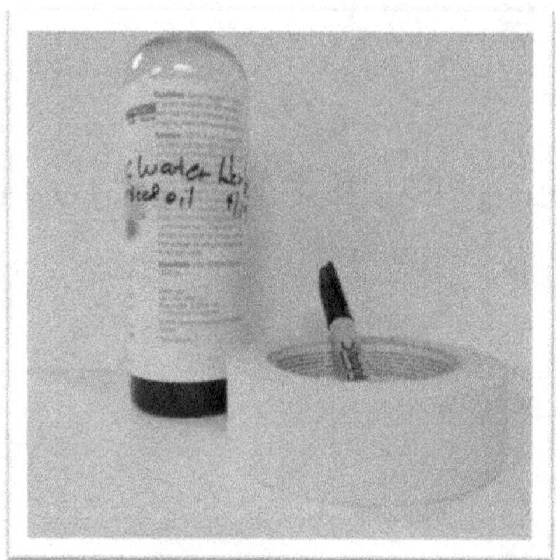

If you are using the whole bottle of oil to make infused propolis oil, pour the infused oil back into the original bottle until you are ready to use it.

Pipettes: sometimes called droppers

Shake, shake, and shake. So how many drops did you really use?

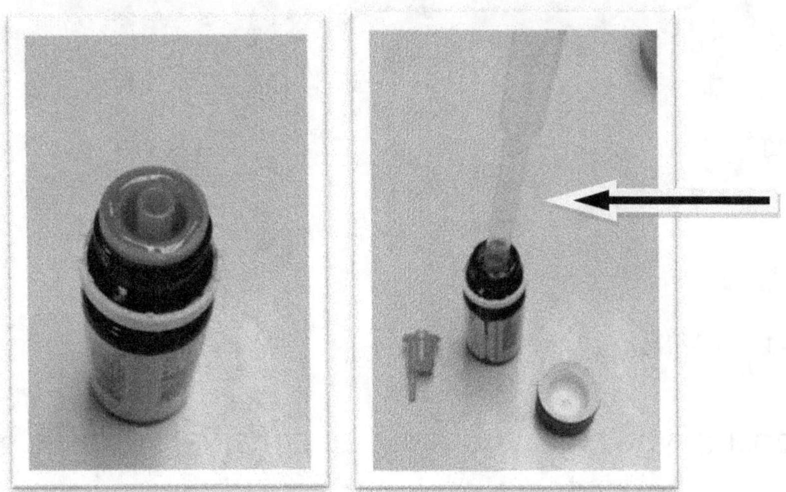

Remove the dropper insert and use a pipette.
You can measure by the drops or ml.
These can be disposed of or cleaned with alcohol for future use.
Use a different pipette for combining different essential oils or clean
with alcohol before going from one bottle to the next.

Weighing liquids:

When weighing the liquid on your scales as carefully as you can, what if
you get just a few more grams than you need: Use a pipette to easily
remove the extra grams.

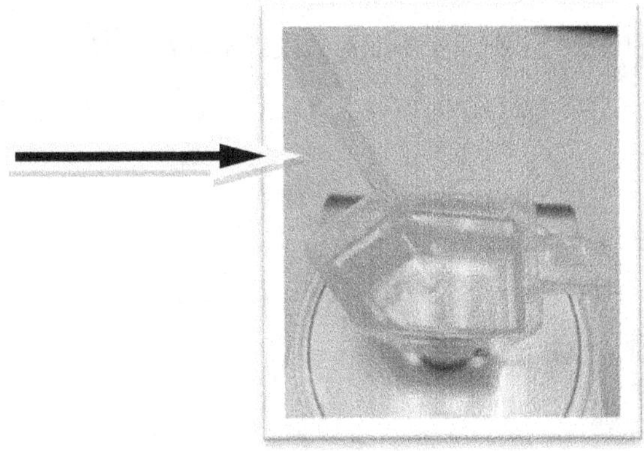

8 Choosing your Oils

When choosing your oils you need to consider, does it have a long shelf life, how is it absorbed by the skin, does it leave a greasy feeling? What are its benefits?

How was it processed?

Is it a seed, a nut or a grain? If you have allergies to nuts than you are certainly going to be allergic to oils made from nuts.

 Definitions:

Unrefined, virgin
These are left in their original state after pressing. They retain more of their beneficial properties and retain their natural flavors and aromas.

Refined:
These oils are refined and filtered to remove impurities. They may have less of their true flavor and aroma.

Cold Pressed:
The seed or nut or fruit is extracted by pressing without chemicals or high heat. The temperature is maintained under 90◦f - 100◦f.
This is considered the best extraction method for maintaining the beneficial properties of the oil.

My Favorite Oils

Almond Oil: Prunus amygdalus dulcis, nut oil

I like to use Almond Oil in my lip balms and ointments used for intimate places.
It is lightweight, anti-inflammatory, moisturizing, nourishing, relieves itching, soothing, high in EFAs and vitamin A and E. It is good for all skin types.
Shortcomings: Will go rancid sooner than coconut oil or olive oil.

Coconut Oil: Cocos nucifera, nut oil

Coconut oil is one of my favorite oils because it has great benefits for the skin and is not likely to go rancid. It is antibacterial, antifungal, anti-inflammatory, antioxidant, cooling, hydrating, moisturizing, nourishing, softening, soothing, UV protective, and high in vitamins A and E.
Its shortcoming is that it is liquid when above 76◦f and becomes solid when under 76◦f.
If it is cold it can become as hard as a rock.
It has to be mixed with other oils and it is very greasy by itself.

Grapeseed Oil: Vitis vinifera, seed oil

I like to use Grapeseed oil in most of my products because it is easily absorbed and does not leave a greasy feeling. It is one of the best oils for lotions meant to go on the face. Grapeseed oil is rich in beta-carotene and vitamins D, C and E.   It contains **essential fatty acids**: perform well in anti-wrinkle trials. **Polyphenols**: anti-inflammatory antioxidants which are known to retard the aging process and prevent acne outbreaks. **Flavonoids OPC**: Biochemical research has found it is rich in Flavonoids OPC that removes free radicals and promotes the restoration of collagen at the cellular level.

Jojoba Jojoba Oil: Jojoba Esters: This is actually a wax from seed and not an oil

I would use Jojoba Jojoba more often if it wasn't so much more expensive than the other oils. It acts as a humectant and creates a protective coating on the skin, keeping in the moisture. It leaves the skin feeling soft without clogging the pores. This oil is the most like the sebum produced by our own skin. Jojoba Jojoba is rich in vitamin E and has a very long shelf life.

Olive oil: Olea europaea, seed oil

Olive oil is the preferred oil for making healing oils from herbs. It has a long shelf life and is considered medium oil. It is anti-inflammatory, anti-bacteria, antioxidant, hydrating, moisturizing, nourishing, reduces itchy skin, softening, soothing, high in EFAs and vitamins E and K.

Sesame Oil: Sesamum indicum, seed oil

An excellent skin emollient that will not stain clothes. It has a large vitamin E content which makes it an excellent antioxidant and gives it a long shelf life. However, it has a distinct aroma which some may not appreciate.

Castor Oil: Ricinus communis, seed oil
Castor oil is thicker than most oils, mild and odorless.
It is high in triglyceride composed of fatty acids. 90% of the acids are ricinoleic acid. It is a natural emollient oil that softens and nourishes the skin. It is used in Castor Oil Packs and can be used to massage into joints and muscles.

Mineral Oil: a petroleum product
All natural oils will eventually go rancid, some sooner than others.
Those that are concerned about using petroleum products and their health will not even consider anything made from petroleum.
Petroleum jelly as the name implies is made from petroleum. Paraffin wax is a petroleum product.

Mineral oil and petroleum jelly will not go rancid and do not harbor bacteria. There are no allergies to petroleum products.
We all grew up with petroleum jelly and baby oil. Baby oil is mineral oil and a synthetic fragrance. Although you may not be allergic to the petroleum jelly, you could be allergic to the synthetic fragrance.

Hospitals will use petroleum jelly and mineral oil because it does not go rancid and will remain more sterile and no concerns with an allergy response. Prescription ointments are made with petroleum jelly.

Mineral oil does not soak into the skin but lies on top providing a barrier. There may be times that you want that barrier, such as preventing a bandage from sticking to a wound or protection from excessive washing of hands or even protection on your lips from the elements.

Natural oils soak into the skin, nourish the skin and go rancid. Your ointments, lip balms, propolis oils will all eventually go rancid using natural ingredients. If you need long time storage you will need to refrigerate these items.

If you are preparing for man-made or natural disasters you might want to consider having some products made with mineral oil for long time storage.

9 Resources for Supplies

Containers and Supplies:

Even though you are buying wholesale, quantity is everything. Buy a small amount and you are not saving much over retail.

I cannot find everything I need at one store. I use:

Bulkapothecary.com

Wholesalesupplyplus.com for the Malibu bottles and the lotion bar tubes

Specialtybottle.com for the tins

Gotoilsupplies.com for the nasal spray bottles

Mountain Rose Herbs.com

Starwest-Botanicals.com: You will need a storefront to purchase wholesale from them.

Drug Emporium will carry many of the cold pressed oils, essential oils, vitamin E, and containers and even beeswax.

Labels:
There are many printing companies to choose from.
I use Avery.com when I need just a few labels or I am experimenting.

To make a few labels at a time, Avery makes it simple to design your labels online with their wide selection of self adhesive labels available at the office supply stores. They have everything from white to craft paper, rounds, ovals and squares.

When you buy your labels be sure and watch if the labels are for a laser printer or an inkjet, of if they are for both.

File folder labels are made to stick to paper and will not remain stuck on glass and plastic.

Avery has templates that have designs on them. I always choose the blank one, because I have too much information to go on the label.
You can insert clip art, photographs or use their limited stock clipart.
I use Art Explosion software for my clip art.

Tip: Mark your printer paper and print a sample before wasting valuable label paper to be sure if your printer is printing on the top side or bottom side.

Watch your office supply sales and stock up.
Avery will also print them for you. www.Avery.com

ABOUT THE AUTHOR

Carolyn Gibson, LMT, Family Herbalist and the Beekeeper's wife and helper, has been a licensed massage therapist since 1996. She fell in love with herbs in the early 70's and has been growing and making herbal remedies since.

Carolyn Gibson and her husband operate Dogwood Gardens Organic Farm since 1991.
Carolyn and Gerald grow wheatgrass and take care of their bee hives.

She teaches how to make herb remedies with beeswax and propolis here on their farm.
Her classes are a "hands on" workshop. Students take home the remedies that they make and written instructions to take home.

Contact Carolyn at:
Carolyngibson1951@gmail.com

Keep up with her classes at:
www.FamilyGuidetoHerbs.com

Check out her many books at Amazon.com